SEW CHIFFON
and
OTHER SHEERS

*Exciting New Ways
to Sew Beautiful Woven Sheers*

—— ❧ ——

Elizabeth Croy

First Edition

B. L. Frame Publishing

SEW CHIFFON AND OTHER SHEERS

Exciting New Ways to Sew Beautiful Woven Sheers

Elizabeth Croy

Copy Editor: Richard W. Croy

Technical Director: James B. Croy

Cover: Schwalb Creative Communications Inc.

Acknowledgements: Barbara Bowman, Jack Buckley, Hal Childs, Clotilde, William E. Croy, Margaret Islander, Steve Kaufman, Patricia Morrow, Judith O'Brien, Mary Mulari, Carolyn Payne and John Starr.

Library of Congress Catalog Card Number 90-84987
ISBN 0-9627879-5-7

B. L. Frame Publishing

CONTENTS

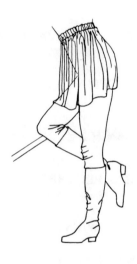

YES, YOU CAN

Every spring and every holiday-time sheer fabrics burst on the fashion scene heralding the special change of activities. We welcome the excitement in this shift in atmosphere and the part our clothes play in it.

Some seasons it seems almost every type garment you can imagine shows up in a fashion magazine or in store window made in a sheer. Other seasons the designers are more restrained in their presentations. Yet, year after year, sheers are on the fashion scene.

This book has been designed to help you produce just what you want, whether it's a voile shirt over a tank top or the most formal gown. When you can't find a flattering pattern designed for a sheer, you're taken by the hand and guided through the intricacies of using your favorite pattern. No leaving you dangling when a procedure is half finished, wondering what you do next.

Do you ever see an old movie and marvel that the leading lady looks stunning in her chiffon ensemble? A case in point is Susan Hayward wearing a stunning chiffon and crepe creation in The Honey Pot, a film made many years ago. Although you may think she had a perfect figure, that's unlikely. Every woman has figure faults. She looks wonderful because the gown is a flattering color, the cut of the gown hides her imperfections and emphasizes her good points, the style is classic and the fabric is timeless.

You can do the same for yourself using your talent, time and sewing machine. It's not free but it cost a lot less money than a garment you buy which doesn't fit and isn't your best color. We've all come home from a shopping expedition with a garment that was wrong for us. We wondered why we bought it, but on reflection, we knew it was the best we could do. This book frees you from wasting your money on clothes you never wear.

Every woman feels she looks her best in a certain type ensemble. You don't like floating draperies? You like narrow skirts? You're the tailored type? Stick with what you think makes you look your best. When you feel you look good you carry yourself with a special self-assurance and things go better in every department. You can still shift your usual appearance just a bit by using different fabrics than you do ordinarily. This is mentioned throughout the book.

You will notice that not many types of sheers are called by name. One year a certain one flashes into the limelight, hovers there a season or two and then another shoots into prominence to replace it. It is our hope you will keep this book for years to help you sew. If you can't find the sheer you're after by a certain name, you'll find, instead, an intriguing first cousin.

In a similar vein, don't concern yourself with such things as skirt lengths, lapel widths and styles that you see in the illustrations. Those things change; good sewing practices don't.

The arrangement of information in this book is logical and easy to use. Subject matter is grouped together by chapters, such as Sewing Above the Waist. Sometimes you are directed to a system demoted by the **#** sign in the chapter you are reading. These are in numerical order, of course. If it's in another chapter, you're told which one. Whether a description is accompanied by one picture or many, it is numbered accordingly as to chapter and location. For instance, if you're told to see 3-6, step 1, you turn to chapter 3 and the picture-group is the sixth in the chapter. Step 1 is the first picture or procedure in that group. When you read about it, the text is nearby and carries the same numbers. The illustrations give visual support to the written word.

A surprising fact emerged after this book was written. Although it is supposed to be for sheers, it turns out to be a fine guide for any silky, slippery fabric that causes problems on the cutting-board and at the sewing machine. You will turn to it time after time when you cut out and sew linings, silky blouses, and other squirmy fabrics-- as well as the sheers.

This book will be one of your best friends in the sewing room.

1

THE MUSLIN GARMENT

A special event usually sets your head spinning wondering what you will wear. When your heart is set on chiffon you may be in for a rude shock to find there aren't many selections in the big pattern books. Perhaps your most flattering styles aren't represented at all. However, some are available and you may find just what you need. Remember, for your first sheer garment, simpler is better. Chapter 2 helps you handle a pattern that's not specifically designed for these see-through beauties. No matter which route you go -- use a pattern designed for a sheer, or adapt one of your own favorites -- you will need to alter the pattern so it fits perfectly. You will make a trial garment in unbleached muslin. In our example we use a dress (fig. 1-1) because it faces most issues. This

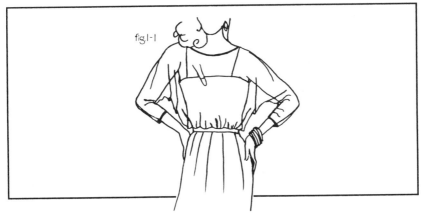

fig.1-1

alteration business is presented now because you cannot proceed even with a commercially designed chiffon pattern until the fit is correct. Perhaps you have heard women say they don't have time to fool with this step but it is essential.

Muslin

Buy unbleached muslin, the old standby for trial sewing, in the lightest weight available. At the mill-end store you can often find a most satisfactory quality that is very little heavier than cheesecloth and duplicates chiffon's flexibility. If you can't find this, buy any plain color cotton in the most lightweight and softest you can find. The paler the color the better.

Use a stiffer trial fabric if you plan to make your garment in a cloth such as organza.

Although in theory you can use any cotton for the trial dress -- even patterned fabric -- this isn't strictly true. The weight of the cotton may be perfect, but, not only is the pattern distracting when you try to fit the dress, you must also hunt all over to find your alteration marks. A plain dress fabric of good quality in your favorite color, even if it is just something left over from another project, is equally diverting. In the back of your mind is the nagging thought that you should make something wearable from such nice material.

Forget it.

Use unbleached muslin so you can focus your attention on the job at hand: to alter the trial dress to fit your individual figure.

Prepare Pattern

You will need to make a few minor changes in your pattern if it isn't designed for sheer sewing (chs. 2 and 3) before you can cut and fit the muslin. Simply turn back to these earlier pages when you are ready for the trial dress. But even with a special chiffon pattern you need to follow these paragraphs for sewing success. Time spent now will avoid tears later.

Have the skirt pattern at least 3 in. longer than the estimated finished length. This is important. If you are taller than average, tape extra paper to the bottom of the skirt patterns. If you plan to use the deep hem, the skirt length should extend beyond the lower edge twice the depth of the hem plus 3 in. To refresh your memory, use the deep hem only for the straight skirt -- pleated, gathered or plain -- without flare.

If there are certain alterations you always make in a pattern, such as the correction for dowager's hump, make them now.

Your weight may change and the next time you use the pattern you will need different alterations. If you want to preserve the original, make a facsimile for each piece. When you look up facsimile in the dictionary it says "an exact copy." No taking it to the copy shop because some machines distort the size.

Make Facsimile

Use your favorite method to reproduce the pattern pieces or use the one that follows.

You need semi-transparent drafting paper, available at big office equipment and artist and drafting supply stores. It always comes in rolls 36 in. wide and sometimes narrower. Buy the thinnest, cheapest type possible because you don't need the high quality architects use. Besides sharing it with a friend, you can saw in half for two 18-in. rolls, quite useful providing you don't have wide pattern pieces.

Select one pattern piece, press with a warm iron and place it with the writing side upward on a piece of white poster board or your big cutting board. No need for pins to hold in place if you spray the back corners of the pattern first with a tiny squirt of Pattern-Sta. Place the drafting paper, cut somewhat larger, on top using a dot of Pattern-Sta at each corner. Or, use pins to hold.

You will have no difficulty seeing all marks through the thin paper. Use a pencil to trace all pertinent lines -- straight of grain, notches, information dots -- everything you need to cut and sew the dress

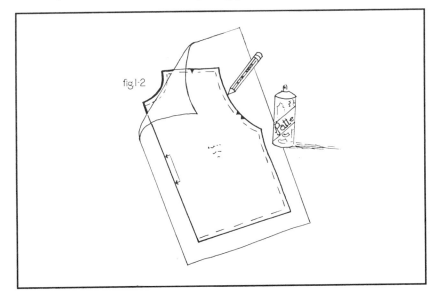

fig.1-2

(fig. 1-2). Aim for accuracy, because even 1/16 inch makes a difference if it is repeated several times. Use a straightedge to draw all straight lines. Before you separate the two layers, be sure to label the facsimile. Set aside this copy but do not cut out. Do the next pattern piece.

Follow the same procedure for the lining.

Cut and Sew the Muslin

Cut out the muslin dress the same length as the pattern with its extra 3 in., making all necessary construction marks with the tracing wheel and tracing paper. Cut it on the straight of grain, just as you will the actual fashion cloth. Adjust the machine to sew about 6 stitches per in. Since you won't bother about facings, you can cut away seam allowances around outside edges of collar and along buttoned openings. But install a zipper or sew on buttons and cut slits for buttonholes so you can accurately test the fit. You need sharply contrasting thread such as red and, because you aren't sewing for permanence or strength, old thread you see in those sale baskets -- even rotten thread -- will do.

Follow the same procedure for the lining.

The Fit, Pins, Pen and Notebook

You may think two layers of muslin at the bodice, and possibly three in the skirt, will be too bulky to judge the fit. But you use a different approach. You make the dress and lining separately and alter each to fit individually before you join them. Take another look at the dress with dolman sleeves; the dress bodice is loose while the lining is somewhat snug (fig. 1-1). You have two entirely different kinds of garments to fit and if you tried to do the fitting while they were sewn together you could tell nothing about either one.

Put on the muslin that represents the dress and fit it first. The example has no set-in sleeves, but if it did you would check for the correct armhole seam placement. (Always try to use a pattern that is the correct size in the neck because it is difficult to alter.) Unless you usually have to shorten the bodice a great deal, don't make any adjustments there just yet. If the sleeve has a cuff, baste it in place because you will sew the cuff to the sleeve before you install the sleeve in the armhole when you make the actual dress. Therefore, the sleeve length must be exactly right in this trial garment.

If you don't feel competent at fitting, get help from a friend who is good at it.

The black felt-tipped pen with a medium point is perfect for marking changes and instructions directly on the muslin dress. You may need to print such things as "stop here," "taper to nothing" or "gather to here." You may even use different colors of pens for different kinds of instructions. The muslin being off-white or cream colored will show the pen marks clearly. Have your notebook at hand to jot down information and to supplement pen marks and pins. You will find this method so satisfactory that once you've tried it you will want to use it for every special garment you make.

Sew the changed muslin trial according to your pins, pen marks and notations.

Repeat for the lining. But a word about the lining. If it is quite different from the dress as in the illustration, yes, you need to try it in muslin. But if you use the same pattern pieces, or they are cut the same size, (compare the patterns) you need not bother.

When the fit of each garment is satisfactory when tried separately, baste them together at the waistline (in this case) and examine them critically as a unit. If the chiffon bodice is blouson, did you accidentally remove the extra length at the waist seam? Is the lining still correct to allow such blousing? Don't worry if a gathered area appears a little bulky in the muslin. It will be satisfactory when you sew it in the thin cloth. If the outer garment is a stiffer sheer, then you must take note and decide if the pattern is correct for such fabric. Always consider the fashion fabric.

A word of caution: do not over-fit. The designer built in a certain "style" which you can easily destroy if your efforts are too energetic.

Length

When you are satisfied with the sewn-together muslins, mark with the pen on the dress below the proposed hemline as follows: C.F. on the center front seam (or where one would be), R.S. on *your* right side seam,

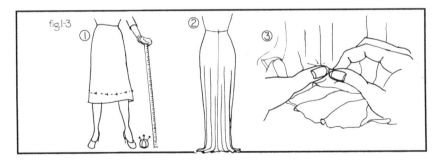

C.B. at the center back seam and L.S. on your left side seam. Figure 1-3, belt the dress if required, step into the correct shoes and **1.** have your friend mark your chosen length for a street-length dress. **2.** If it is a floor-length gown, **3.** mark it where it touches the floor. Cut off the excess fabric and lay the strip aside carefully. You may suspend the dress in a doorway, or such, and cut off the skirt and lining the same length.

Why do you cut off the muslin?

The purpose is threefold: you can manage the next pattern step, you can accurately judge the appearance of the garment in its finished length and you have the dress to try on and refer to later.

Lay the cut-off piece of muslin on the bottom of the corresponding part of the pattern (fig. 1-4) matching the bottom edges. **1.** Mark at the newly cut edge. **2.** Below this mark you add 3 in. Cut off the pattern on this last line and discard any pattern below. This 3 in. is your insurance policy against ravelings and miscalculations. As you gain experience, you can add a little less extra cloth.

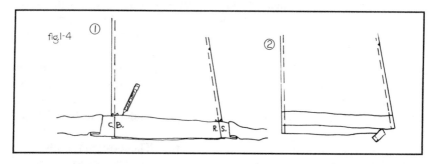

Transfer the Changes

Make sure every alteration, shown in fig. 1-5, step **1**, is clearly marked on the muslin with the pen. Carefully rip apart the altered sections and press gently with a dry iron with the grain so you don't distort the shape.

On the cutting-board place the pattern (or facsimile) of one part of the dress that you have to alter, and over it pin the altered portion of the muslin dress, matching centers and edges exactly. Push a few big-headed pins through to the cutting-board to hold in place. **2.** Slip in transfer paper, business side down against the pattern, and run the tracing wheel over all the changes following the pen marks, pins and notebook jottings.

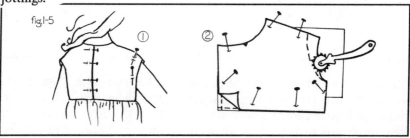

Repeat for all the other changed pieces. Then, adjust the seam allowances to correspond to these new lines. Don't forget to alter touching or matching places such as facings or adjoining seams.

Remember that you didn't cut out the traced pattern pieces -- the facsimiles? Now you may need the extra paper. Suppose you want just a little more ease over the hip area. You can add the amount where needed without having to tape on more paper.

Erase all original lines that are no longer appropriate. Use these new pattern pieces as you proceed.

Little Girls

When you sew for little girls, your task is much simpler. You need to choose a pattern that fits correctly at the neck and then adjust shoulder seams, armholes, waist and length, just as you usually do. There's a lot less fine tuning. Still, you want the dress to look like it came from an exclusive children's shop, not a bargain store.

DO NOT CHEAT ON THESE STEPS. You may think it takes too much time, but you are wrong. You must sew sheer cloth correctly the first time to prevent that shopworn look. If you try to baste, try on, fit, stitch, try on, rip, -- on and on, the cloth looks used. With this muslin method you can sew the most costly cloth with confidence. None of those uneasy feelings, hoping it will fit and look right.

Take some extra time at this point to alter the trial garment and lining to fit perfectly and then change the pattern to meet your special requirements. No amount of fine sewing can overcome a poor fit.

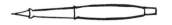

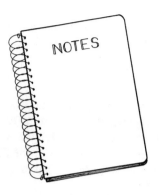

2

This Isn't What I Need   THE PATTERN DOESN'T SAY CHIFFON

What do you do when you can't find a pattern you want that's especially designed for chiffon or another sheer? Are you doomed to sew a style that doesn't suit your figure?

No.

Actually, this very lack in the pattern books can be a blessing in disguise. The first rule in sewing for yourself is to pick a style that does flattering things for *you*. Nothing can be as important as this -- not fabric, not color, nothing. The wrong style, no matter how perfect otherwise, can't do nice things for your appearance.

Although many styles can be handled one way or another so you can sew them in a sheer, for your first such garment choose a simple style. The fewer details and the fewer seams, the more success you will have. However, this chapter covers them all. If you are a very experienced seamstress, you can just forge ahead because all general types of garments are on these pages.

There are many exciting non-traditional methods in ch. 9 for using chiffon, Georgette and other sheers. For those, keep reading. However, if you want to try a more informal method, such as using chiffon over knits or making a brief chiffon skirt to wear over a leotard, skip these first three chapters for now. Come back to them when you are interested in a conventional garment from see-through cloth and note the pattern changes you may need. Read applicable parts of the other chapters, however, so you can sew with ease and make your garment completely practical.

CHIFFON AND OTHER SHEERS

What's in a Name?

Don't be put off because chiffon is mentioned much of the time instead of naming other sheers. Often, it's for brevity. In the end, you must consider the sheerness of the cloth and the flexibility. For example, some organza is extremely sheer and has the same requirements about lining for concealment as chiffon. But think about the stiffness. That makes it unfit for patterns that are perfect for a very drapable Georgette. By the same token, the softness of chiffon makes it unsuitable for details such as self- supporting puffed sleeves unless you put a stiffening inside. Touch and appearance help you decide if the sheer and the pattern make a good team. If you are uncertain, ask an experienced salesperson or a friend to help you.

Understand Your Needs

Before you can buy your fabrics, you have to know just what you need. This chapter helps you identify lining and underskirt requirements and the next chapter helps you make those necessary adjustments and change simple patterns if required. It's pretty heady stuff! Perhaps you didn't think you could ever do such things, but you can do it easily if you follow the directions and pictures.

Sometimes you need to provide yourself with simple basic patterns which you may already have. They are now in the big books, and some are listed in the back of this book. You can also take advantage of your friends' pattern collections and patronize garage sales and the like.

THE CHALLENGES OF SHEERS

What are some of the differences between sewing with ordinary opaque cloth and a sheer? For one thing, with a very sheer cloth you can see through it to whatever is underneath. No secrets here! Better be sure that every bit of underwear you display is something you want on parade for all to see. For example, should the shoulder area be covered by only the sheer, show only one set of shoulder straps. You may wear a strapless bra under the camisole or you may put wide straps on the upper set that will hide the straps below. You can cover regular bra straps with lining fabric and then invisibly sew the finished lining garment -- without straps -- to the bra at the point where bra and straps join; then tack liner dress and bra together other places, such as under the arms and at the cleavage. But you must do something because it is an unpleasant fact of life: more than one set of shoulder straps seen through sheer cloth makes you look untidy. For this reason you need to know about mounting.

Mounting

What is mounting? As mentioned in ch. 1, after you cut out a

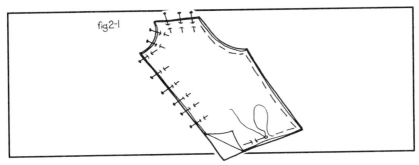

fig2-1

piece of fashion fabric, baste it to an exactly matching piece of lining (in this case) and thereafter handle the unit as a single piece of cloth (fig. 2-1). This is very useful for the woman whose bra straps cut into her shoulders or who cannot wear a strapless bra. If the bodice of your sheer has normally placed armholes, you may mount the chiffon bodice on the lining fabric and proceed. If the bodice has a yoke you can mount the yoke.

Workmanship

Another difference is that through a very sheer cloth you also see every seam, every dart, every construction detail and just how well you did each! Again, no secrets. No hiding sloppy work. You'll read about sewing techniques later, but you need to know about darts now because there is an optional change you may want to make in your pattern.

Darts

The perfect pattern for a sheer has no visible darts and few seams. Since this isn't always possible, we need to know how to deal with darts to change them to another form or to make them unobjectionable. If there are darts you absolutely can't do without -- when substitute shaping won't do -- then you must use them, of course. The alteration for a dowager's hump might be a case in point.

Placket

Another difference is you may not have to bother with the ever-troublesome zipper. The cloth bound-placket, surprisingly easy to do and quite successful, is perfect for sheerest cloth if the garment is not tightly fitted. You have to be a contortionist, almost, to fasten it up the back where it's usually placed, but it is lovely.

Concealment

Yet another difference is a two-parter: while you want to display parts of your person and perhaps some fancy underwear, you want privacy other places. The concealing layer you need in some areas is the lining;

it goes next to your skin unless it's faced. In the traditional type chiffon garment, the lining and any underskirts hang free from the waist, whether it is high or low. We deal with the lining later.

Underskirts for the Wide Skirt

If there is an underskirt, it is directly under the chiffon skirt and cut narrower. It goes on top of the lining. Although it is not always appropriate, when it is used, it is the unseen glorifier. Or, more accurately, the *unnoticed* glorifier.

If the skirt is gathered or flared, a chiffon underskirt adds a luxurious touch. Strangely enough, its presence is not noticed, but its absence makes the dress look spare and cheap. Under a bouffant gown (fig. 2-2) it is possible to have several chiffon underskirts (always slightly

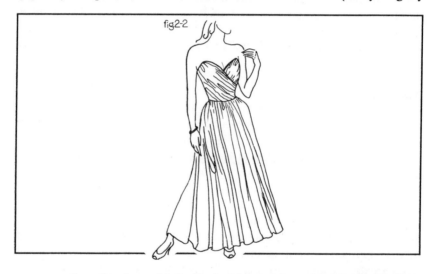

fig2-2

narrower than the dress skirt) all of which need not be exactly the same fabric. If the gown is silk, you can make some layers from rayon chiffon which must also go to the drycleaners and has a similar hand. Or, you may need a slightly stiffer sheer for some layers and then make a lower layer of taffeta. (Last of all comes the lining layer.) Needless to say, the colors must be correct. This "debutante" type gown may not be the vogue right now. If not, it is bound to return; fashions always repeat themselves.

Underskirt for the Narrow Skirt

What about the "straight" skirt? While you understand that the wide chiffon skirt requires more than one chiffon layer, you may overlook the narrow skirt in this department. Many expensive chiffon dresses have this subtle enhancement regardless of the skirt width. There are times when the chiffon underskirt may be undesirable or unnecessary -- when the lining carries the design, is lace and the like.

However, even in the above situations you may need to use the extra layer when the chiffon is ultra thin. An example is the lining made from a particularly bold, colorful pattern covered by a very sheer chiffon. Although you can see there is a film over your arms, unfortunately the print jumps out visually beyond the sheer and from any distance at all it looks as if you are wearing a printed jumper over a chiffon garment. This phenomenon is accentuated if the lining has a camisole or halter top. This is NOT the effect you want. There are several solutions, but one is to use two layers of chiffon for the body of the chiffon garment instead of one.

You probably won't have this problem with a more opaque cloth such as voile, so here's a good rule to remember: the more sheer the cloth, the more it benefits from an extra layer of a sheer underneath.

Lining

The lining serves two practical purposes. First, it provides concealment as required. An evening dress you wear in public needs a much different lining than the peignoir you wear in the privacy of your home. Second, the lining provides a foundation against which the chiffon rests and complements the design of the garment. A gown with a bouffant skirt requires a lining with more body than the gown that is soft or flowing.

For several reasons the lining skirt is most narrow of all. For one, when you sit, the narrower width prevents the lining from showing at the hem below the sheer skirt. For another, the narrower width keeps it and all skirt layers over it from "walking" between your legs as you move, a most annoying occurrence that has you plucking surreptitiously at the side of your dress. Even for a long skirt the lining usually need be no wider than 72 in. at the hemline, depending on your height and weight, of course.

Regardless of hem width, you must cut the lining generously enough over the hips -- only a smidgen less than the dress itself -- so that when you sit it doesn't ride up noticeably higher than the chiffon dress. Along the same line, don't cut the lining on the bias unless the chiffon skirt is also bias and about the very same width.

To Sum Up Skirt Layers The sheer dress skirt is the widest; the underskirt, if any, is somewhat narrower, and the lining skirt is the narrowest of all.

One last word: unless you use a totally separate lining garment, fasten the lining at waist, underarms or near chest area so that when you raise your arms the skirt lining won't hang below skirt hem.

WHAT DOES YOUR PATTERN NEED?

Now that you have a firm grasp on the handling of underskirts and linings, you want to apply the knowledge to your own pattern. Here's how to use the following paragraphs.

Have a picture of your sheer garment at hand, perhaps the pattern envelope. Notice the characteristics you can put into certain slots, such as a flared skirt without pleats or gathers, or a set-in band. Ask yourself some pertinent questions. Does it have darts you need to handle? If it is a coat or blouse, do you already have the separate lining garment or must you sew or buy it? If it has a yoke, do you want it lined to hide bra straps or do you want the unlined, bare-shoulder look? Next, glance through the categories of the special paragraphs and put check marks by those which apply and a paper clip at the top of such pages.

As an example, suppose fig. 2-3 is a picture of your dress pattern. The bodice has a yoke with a collarless neckline, and normally placed

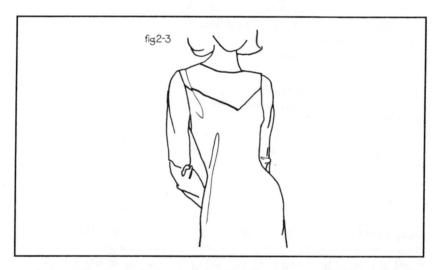

fig 2-3

armholes with closely fitted sleeves without gathers at the top. There is no waistline and you intend to wear the dress unbelted. You study the pattern picture, think about the occasions when you will wear the dress, and decide you want to use plain colored dark chiffon over a plain lining. You like the bare-shouldered look so the chiffon will appear as filmy and delicate as possible.

You glance through the special paragraphs, look at the illustrations and see that you need no patterns other than those that come in the pattern envelope, but that #4 gives information about their slight modification for lining and underskirt patterns. You use check marks and paper clips as future references to the applicable sections. You only need pay attention to these paragraphs at the moment and follow their instructions. However, you will have a firmer understanding of lining requirements if you scan all of them.

The garments in the following illustrations are deliberately simple so you can concentrate on the principal characteristics being featured. Numbers (#) refer to paragraph in the **next** chapter.

DART ADJUSTMENT AND
LINING AND UNDERSKIRT REQUIREMENTS

SHOULDER, UNDERARM AND WAIST DART (fig. 2-4)

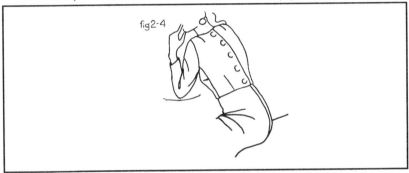

fig2-4

You can change many shoulder, underarm and waistline darts in sheer cloth, to be less noticeable by following #1. Darts are not quite as noticeable if the area is mounted.

DRESS WITH SEPARATE LINING (fig. 2-5)

Almost without exception this sheer dress has no waistline, few pattern pieces and is a straightforward design such as the caftan or simple shift. The lining is a plain garment -- no waistline and few pattern pieces -- which you construct as a separate dress and wear underneath the outer dress. You may choose any shape you like across its top, such as built-up shoulders or straight across, as long as it looks appropriate under the sheer dress and enhances your figure. It should not have elaborate fitting seams because they will detract from the upper garment. It follows your body lines but does not fit tightly.

If the outer garment is rather opaque, make the lining dress out of matching lining or another appropriately colored plain fabric. But, if you use a plain chiffon for the outer garment, you can make the lining dress out of a print or have a special design on the front of the lining skirt, such as sequins or sparkling rhinestones. Should you decide to mount chiffon on the lining dress, an elegant touch when the upper dress is sheerest chiffon, remember this when you add up yardage for your shopping list.

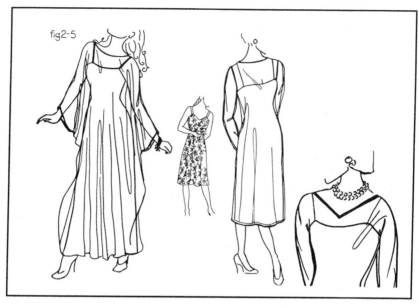

fig2-5

You will find the under-dress in the big books in the lingerie section or in the simple-to-sew section. Should you decide to widen the lining dress slightly to be more appropriate under the loose garment, see #2 and #3.

SHEER COAT, SEPARATE GARMENT UNDERNEATH (fig. 2-6)

This totally separate coat may be short, long, freeflowing, clinched at the waist, hooked at strategic places in the bodice like the oldfashioned redingote; but it isn't buttoned. Besides a plain color, the undergarment may be lace or a print, and either a dress or trousers. You don't attach

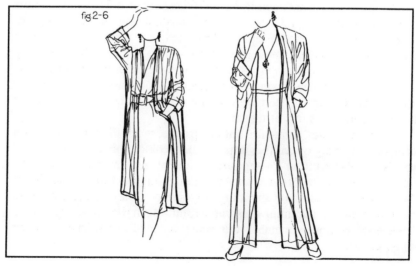

fig2-6

lining to the coat itself.

SHEER SHIRT OR BLOUSE, SEPARATE CAMISOLE UNDERNEATH (fig. 2-7)

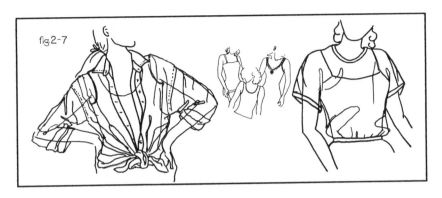

fig 2-7

Make this top from the sheer of your choice of either plain or patterned cloth. As with most separate, unconnected linings, the camisole becomes a part of the design. If you are quite firm and thin, you may make the camisole a closely fitted fancy affair fastened up the front with tiny buttons. In this case your underwear is anything but private. Or, you may choose a completely plain camisole or stretch tank top which you slip over your head before you don the sheer outer garment. Camisole patterns are readily available.

PLAIN SHIFT, PARTIALLY CONNECTED LINING (fig. 2-8)

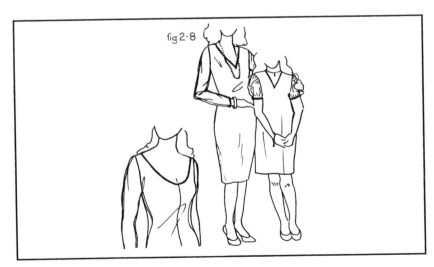

fig 2-8

This simple shift is easy to make but very effective when the style flatters and the fit is good. You may or may not wear it belted. The lining is connected at the neck, armholes and at the placket. If the outer layer is sheer chiffon, you may use a colorful print for the lining if you observe the suggestions you read earlier in this chapter. For the lining use the pattern pieces for the front and back. Read #4 to narrow slightly for the lining skirt and any underskirt, and #3 for notches.

DRESS WITH LINED OR UNLINED YOKE, NO BODICE GATHERS AT YOKE, NO WAIST SEAM (fig. 2-9)

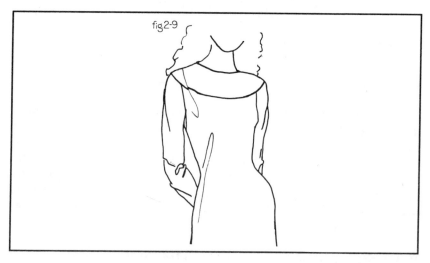

fig 2-9

If the dress is not greatly flared, you can use the dress pattern pieces for any lining as well as for the lush look of another layer of chiffon. See #4 for narrowing for lining and any underskirt, and #3 for notches. If body of garment is greatly flared, use #5 for lining, #6 for underskirt, if belted, and #3 for notches.

DRESS WITH LINED OR UNLINED YOKE, BODICE GATHERED TO YOKE, NO WAIST SEAM (fig. 2-10)

You can use the pattern pieces should you decide to mount and face the yoke. However, this style requires an ungathered lining for the body of the dress unless you are shadow thin. Although chiffon is very sheer and lightweight, the dress will make you look a little heavy if you gather the lining and dress together. (Do not even consider gathering a heavier sheer in with the lining.) You need, therefore, a plain shift pattern with naturally placed armholes, available in the big books. See #5 for lining the body of the dress and #3 for notches.

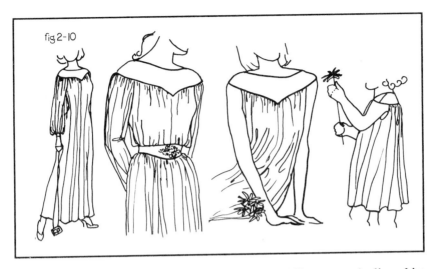

fig. 2-10

If you want an underskirt for a belted shift, use an A-line skirt pattern or follow the directions in #6.

PANTS (fig. 2-11)

Remember that no matter how the trousers are styled, woven sheers don't stretch and pants must be large enough to go over the hips with ease when the placket, if any, is open.

Full, sheer trousers, gathered or pleated to a band at the waist, require a simpler trouser lining with a smaller amount of waist gathers, and cut narrower in the legs below the crotch. Follow #7 and #8.

Wide, flared trouser legs, no gathers or pleats at waist, also require the plain trouser, but with no gathers at waist and cut narrower in the legs. Follow #8.

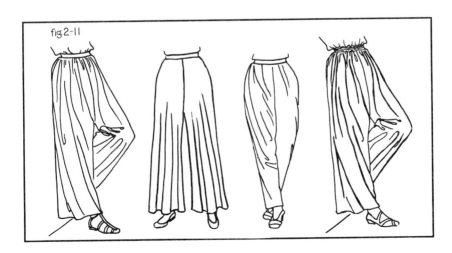

fig. 2-11

Trousers with few if any pleats or gathers may use the pattern narrowing as in #9. (Tight pants are not suitable made in a sheer. Other fabrics are better.)

For trousers sewn to a drawstring band, be sure to test lining pattern ahead of time to be sure it's large enough to pass over the hips with ease. You may narrow the legs a little by following #7 and #8.

Make linings 1/2 to 1 in. shorter (total) in the crotch.

Do NOT under any circumstances, wear only close-fitting knitted pants-liners under chiffon trousers for a lining. You will look as if you are wearing no underwear at all.

GARMENT WITH SET-IN BAND (fig. 2-12)

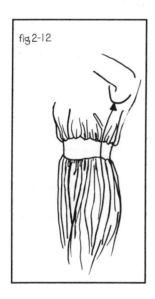
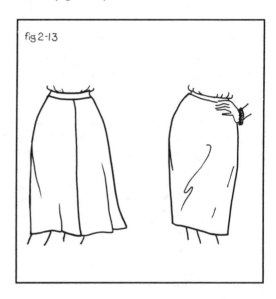

Use the set-in band patterns that come in the pattern envelope for linings, extra layer of chiffon and facings.

SLIM TO MODESTLY FLARED SKIRT, NO PLEATS OR GATHERS (fig. 2-13)

Use the skirt pattern for the lining, narrowing it slightly as suggested in #4. Follow #3 for notches.

SLIM SKIRT WITH ORNAMENTATION (fig. 2-14)

You may need to mount two layers of chiffon to the skirt which you make from lining fabric, and then proceed as the pattern instructs. Or make the skirt solely from crepe. You may also need to sew a

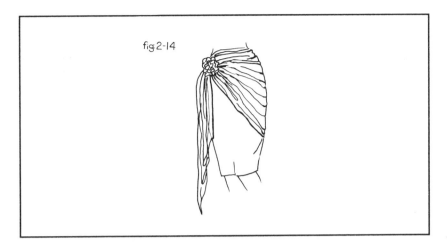

fig 2-14

free-hanging layer of lining inside to the waist seam which will require more lining fabric. This is not for beginners. Remember, wide bias trim like this can stretch with age.

SKIRT WITH GATHERS OR PLEATS (fig. 2-15)

You do not usually gather or pleat a lining in with the sheer because it causes a slightly bulky look. For the plainer lining that you require for the wide-at-the-hem pleated or gathered skirt, use an A-line skirt pattern or a straight skirt pattern, following #2 and #3. The all-around pleated skirt doesn't need an underskirt, but the wide *gathered* skirt does and you can use either #2 or #6, along with #3. For the narrow skirt with ornamental pleats, use the straight skirt pattern using #4, if required, and #3.

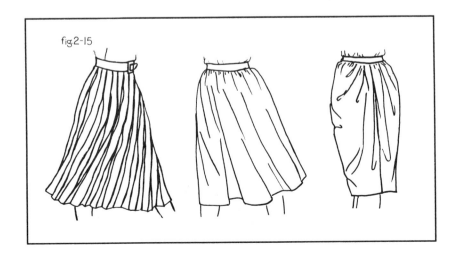

fig 2-15

DEEP HEM (fig. 2-16)

Use the deep hem only on a skirt that has absolutely no flare. Any seams go straight up and down with the grain. For the lining use the A-line skirt pattern cut narrower at the hem than the sheer, or follow #2

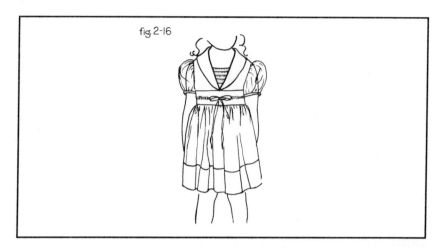

fig. 2-16

and #3. For the underskirt, use #6 for the wide skirt. Don't use the deep hem for lining and underskirt except for children.

FLAT COLLAR (fig. 2-17)

Regardless of the outside shape, this is essentially a flat collar: both the upper and lower layers are cut from exactly the same pattern and, after construction, sewn to the neck. You need no other patterns for lining other than those in the pattern envelope. However, ch. 5, illustrations 5-2 and 5-3, will be helpful.

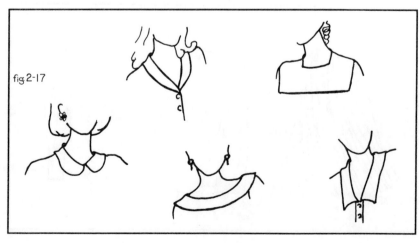

fig 2-17

SHIRT COLLAR (fig. 2-18)

This collar is a standard shirt collar with a band. You will need to add a seam following #11, illustration 1, if the outside edge is on a fold; it must be like a flat collar.

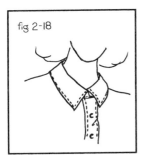 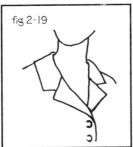 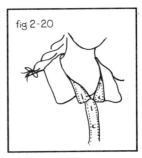

TAILORED COLLAR (fig. 2-19)

If the collar part is the flat collar (above) you need no patterns beyond those in the pattern envelope. For the lapel part, see EXTENDED FRONT FACING, NO SEAM, below.

APPLIED, OR SIMULATED APPLIED, FRONT BODICE OPENING FOR BUTTONS (fig. 2-20)

This front opening appears to have an extra strip topstitched in place for buttonholes. Check 7-8 to see if you can adapt that method for your pattern. If you need to add a seam, follow the ideas in #11.

EXTENDED FRONT FACING, NO SEAM (fig. 2-21)

This is the totally sheer front often used with the sheer collar. It's one of the most simple yet elegant of ways to sew a sheer. You must examine the pattern pieces to know if the facing is attached by a seam. The heavier sheer can *sometimes* use iron-on interfacing and top stitching. You need no additional pattern pieces. However, if you have this type facing (no seam) and want a ruffle, etc., use #11.

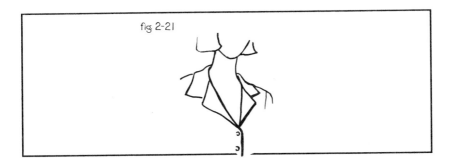

FRONT FACING ATTACHED WITH SEAM (fig. 2-22)

This bodice may or may not have a collar. The simple revers (shown beruffled), formed by folding back a collarless neckline, is an easy answer if you need the appearance of a collar without the difficulty. A collar from fig. 2-21 may look like one from this group on the pattern envelope. The pattern pieces tell the story.

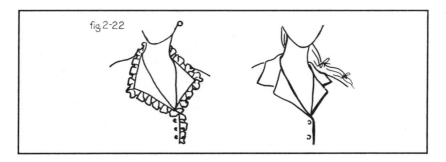

fig. 2-22

V-NECK WITH SEAM IN CENTER FRONT OR SURPLICE CLOSING, BOTH WITH FOLDED-BACK FACING
(fig. 2-23)

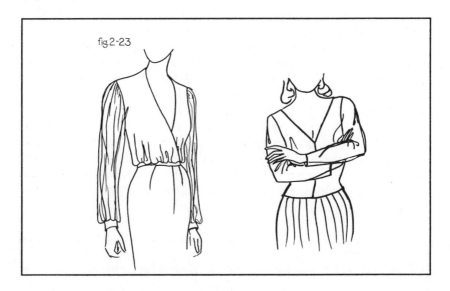

fig. 2-23

The set-in sleeves allow you to mount sheer bodice fabric to lining. (This method isn't suitable for dolman sleeves.) Although you need no additional pattern pieces, cut the sheer 1/2 in. beyond the edge of the facing so you can fold the raw edges out of sight.

SPECIAL NECKLINE TREATMENTS (fig. 2-24)

Be aware that many special necklines when made in opaque cloth appear to be the no-nonsense-lady-lawyer-in-the-courtroom types, but

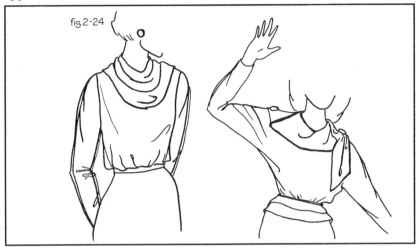

fig. 2-24

when you sew them in a sheer they completely change character. You need no additional pattern pieces.

GOWN WITH STRUCTURED BODICE (fig. 2-25)

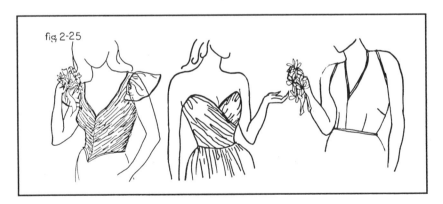

fig. 2-25

This gown may be high or low in the "waistline" and may be bouffant or straight in the skirt. It may be strapless, be sleeveless or have brief sleeves; but the bodice is close-fitting, called structured. It keeps its shape to a marked degree whether you're wearing it or not. This type pattern is usually very good about giving all the special patterns and instructions you need to make a lovely dress. Nevertheless, you will want to mount one or two layers of chiffon on the bodice to keep it from looking cheap. Another good idea is to face the entire close-fitting bodice with a fine quality poly/cotton for wearing comfort. A piping of bias-covered cording marks the waist seam nicely instead of a belt. Any changes you make like this will affect your shopping list.

If the gown isn't strapless and the bodice has waistline and underarm darts to achieve the fit instead of seams, you can have a softer look if you change the darts to shoulder folds, using this changed pattern for the topmost layer of chiffon. The method is similar to that of #1 except you *want* the folds to be noticed. First, fit as designed. Then read #12 for making this change.

DRESS WITH A PARTIAL WAISTLINE, PARTIALLY MOUNTED LINING (fig. 2-26)

This dress has either two principal pattern pieces or a number of long panels. The waistline seam does not go all the way around the body.

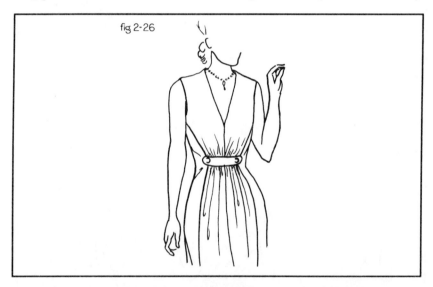

fig 2-26

The bodice has a standard body fit and regular armholes, otherwise it falls into the category of the caftan. In the example, the partial waist seam is in the front although it could be elsewhere. After you are satisfied with the fit of the muslin dress there is an optional change in the lining, #13.

LININGS FOR EMPIRE DRESS (fig. 2-27)

When the skirt is fairly plain and straight, use the skirt pattern in the envelope following #4 and #3, observing the rules in this chapter for lining and underskirts. If the skirt is greatly flared and full, you can follow the principles in #5 for the skirt lining. When the so-called waistline is more or less equidistant from the floor all around, not dipping low in the

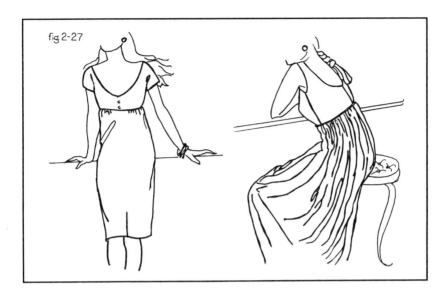

fig 2-27

front or back, use #14 for the 8 gore underskirt pattern -- so practical because the hem hangs correctly year after year, never dropping below the dress hem to expose itself.

You mount sheer to lining for a fitted bodice or use #16 for an attractive lining.

DRESS WITH LOW "WAISTLINE" (fig. 2-28)

When the bodice is simple without much detail, extend it to below where flounce and bodice join for bodice lining. Or, you may use either the simple shift pattern or elongated camisole cut to below bodice/flounce

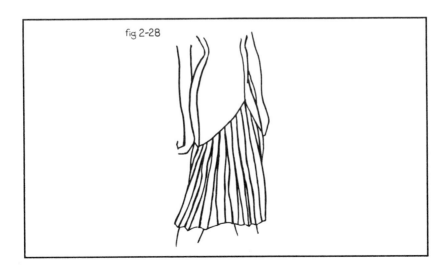

fig 2-28

seam. The flounce, whether pleated, gathered or flared, has its own lining, #15.

DRESS WITH BODICE AND SLEEVES CUT IN ONE
(fig. 2-29)

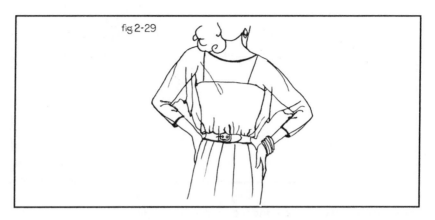

fig 2-29

A special problem arises because the bodice/sleeve unit generally fits loosely while the lining must follow the body lines. You need a camisole-type lining to emphasize the sheerness of the bodice fabric. If you mount the sheer, it will look like a regular fabric because the sleeves will be lined, too. There are a number of ways to handle this problem, all requiring the camisole. #17 gives instructions about adjusting the pattern to open down the back. If your sheer garment opens down the front, one solution is to wear a slip-on camisole cut about blouse length.

CUFFS (fig. 2-30)

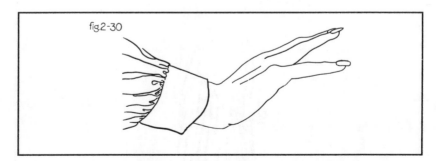

fig 2-30

The cuff pattern, whether one piece or two, requires an adjustment. See #18.

3

What's Behind It All? UNDERSKIRTS AND LINING PATTERNS

The preceding chapter tells you what type lining and underskirts you need for each category of garment. This chapter gives you the numbered paragraphs to follow. Remember, the muslin that represents the sheer must fit first as explained in ch. 1. Read these practical suggestions before you get started on lining and underskirt patterns.

TIPS FOR MAKING YOUR OWN LINING
AND UNDERSKIRT PATTERNS

1. Work on the cutting board so you can push pins into it when required.

2. Make all facsimiles in pencil so you can erase lines when they are no longer appropriate. Don't cut out newly traced facsimile; cut around it leaving plenty of paper so you don't have to paste on more paper if you need to enlarge.

3. In some cases cut away the pattern seam allowance where you will make changes; however, it's helpful to leave a tiny hairline of the broken sewing line. Always make changes on seamline and then add seam allowances.

4. Plan the lining placket in the same location as the sheer.

5. On each pattern piece show the straight of grain, whether or not it goes on the fold and label it.

6. Except for very unusual circumstances, make the lining and underskirts on the straight of grain.

7. Add seam allowances where necessary using a solid line for cutting line.

8. Mark notches (and use them) so matching seams come out the same length.

9. Make the lining shift in muslin or other thin cotton. Fit and try with the muslin dress so you can make any adjustments necessary. Since sheer sleeves are unlined, don't line them in muslin.

10. The side seam of any lining or underskirt should hang from the waist straight down toward the floor and must be corrected if it doesn't. For example, if side seam swings toward the front, pinch out a bit of cloth at the back near the waist seam midway between center back and side seam until side seam hangs down straight toward floor. Trim pinched-up amount from back waist making a deeper curve.

#1 SHOULDER, UNDERARM OR WAIST DART (fig. 3-1)

The small back shoulder dart is used as an example.

1. On the facsimile, mark points 2 in. or less on either side of the dart stitchlines on the shoulder seamline. (The bigger the dart the wider the space on either side.) Cut away the seam allowance between the marks. Starting at the marks, draw lines to the dart point, and then draw about two more on each side and number each. By cutting on the original stitch lines to the point of the dart, the triangle of the dart will fall away.

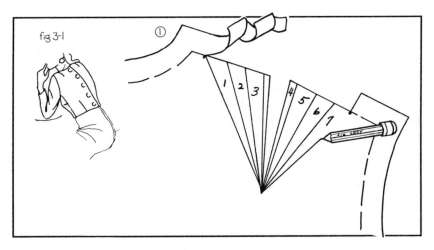

fig 3-1

2. Slip a piece of paper under the entire dart area. Cut on one of the two end lines you drew stopping 1/32 in. short of the point. Draw together the original dart so the edges touch. Hold with pins until you can secure its length with Scotch tape.

A new opening will appear where you made the cut. Slash on all the newly made lines, stopping a hair short of the dart point. If you should cut through and separate a piece, hold its point in place with a big-headed pin. Distribute the space evenly among all the little pieces, holding them with pins and then Scotch tape all in place. The area resembles a little fan. **3.** Even this edge with a pencil, cutting off only the very tips of the fan so the shoulder seam is gently rounded. Add correct seam allowance.

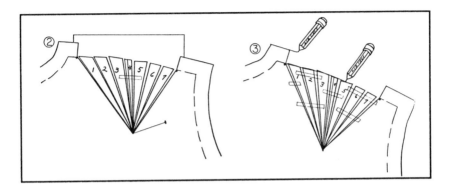

When you sew the muslin, substitute this new pattern, ease the back shoulder in to the front and make any slight adjustment necessary. Use this principal when you need to eliminate any dart.

The Big Dart (fig. 3-2)

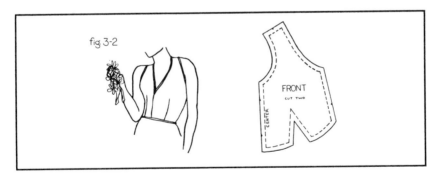

fig 3-2

FRONT
CUT TWO

This applies to the type seen in the large under-the- bust fitting dart. Occasionally, it is the long dart that appears to be a seam in the pattern picture. Do not attempt to ease in this large dart. Sew and finish a special way. See 6-14 and 7-15.

#2 HOW TO WIDEN A GARMENT SLIGHTLY (fig. 3-3)

A slim lining may be perfect in every other way except for being a bit narrower in the skirt than needed. Add a little extra width to the side seams only; the center front and center back always remain on the straight of grain. Decide how much wider you need the entire finished skirt at the hem and divide by 4. Remember, the short lining skirt need be no wider than about 60 in. and the long lining dress 75 or 80 in. Three in. should be the maximum you will add to any one pattern piece at the hem -- that would be 12 inches addition altogether. If the hip size gives you enough ease so the skirt doesn't ride up too much, start the addition near the waist area.

1. If the hips can use a little more space, start addition just under the side-seam bust dart (or where one would be). Put a dot on the seamline where you start. Gently curve the seam through the waist area and then use a straightedge to continue to the correct addition at the hem. Measure down the front to the dot, taking out for the dart. **2.** Mark on the back the same amount. Repeat the addition for the back starting at the dot. **3.** Add correct seam allowances.

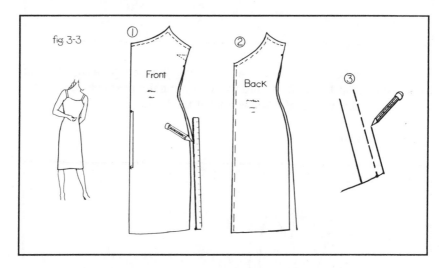

#3 How to Notch Matching Seams (fig. 3-4)
    You need to imitate the notches on the commercial pattern that enable you to match seams and have them the same length. Make several random notches on the new seam allowance of one pattern piece -- it doesn't matter which -- and lay it face up on the cutting board. **1.** Place the joining pattern piece face up on top. Superimpose starting dots and pierce them with a pin. If the seams have the same curve, make them the same length. However, because the front and back of the female body curve differently, the patterns may have a different swing. You will be able so see clearly through the transparent paper. Follow down the stitchline from dots for as far as the seams are exactly together. At the point where they diverge, pierce the stitchline with another pin. **2.** Remove the pin above and swing the upper pattern to follow the stitchline of lower pattern. Repeat if necessary . Two or three such operations should easily take you to the place where the seam straightens out.

Mark notches in upper pattern as you come to them. Cut upper pattern the same length as lower pattern.

Alternately, you can use a spline (a flexible curve) to measure and mark notches.

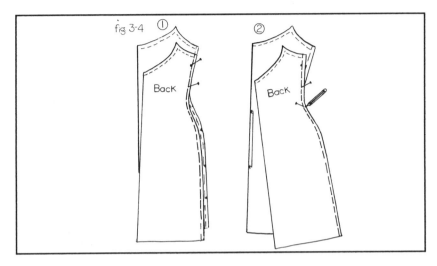

#4 HOW TO NARROW A GARMENT SLIGHTLY (fig. 3-5)

1. Decide the total amount of narrowing you want from the pattern you use as a guide. Divide by 4 and make a dot this amount in from the side seam at the hem to front skirt pattern. Start the narrowing just below the fullest part of the area, such as just below the hip. Join line to hem dot. **2.** Add seam allowances and repeat for the back. Use #3 for notches. (Remember that the underskirt is a little narrower than the sheer and the lining is narrowest of all.)

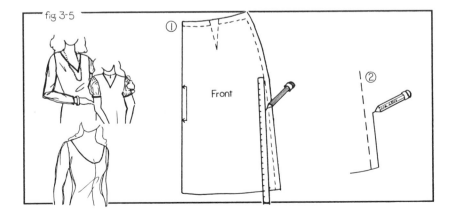

#5 HOW TO MAKE A PLAIN LINING FOR A GATHERED AREA

In this example, the bodice is gathered to a yoke and the dress opens down the back. Mark center backs and center front with machine stitches. Should the lining pattern have waistline fitting darts, use them or not depending on the desired fit. If the yoke is low on the bodice you may be able to use the shift with a camisole top. Wear a strapless bra if you want the bare-shoulder look.

Muslin Shift (fig. 3-6) The shift should have normally placed armholes. **1.** If your pattern was made to accommodate shoulder pads, you may need to take a bit off the outer shoulder seam, removing less as you approach neck, and possibly trim the armholes a little. **2.** The ideal body fit is smooth, not tight. **3.** Put on the lining muslin and pin the opening together. Should you plan to belt the garment, tie a string around your waistline and mark this line with the pen. Put on over it the muslin that represents the sheer.

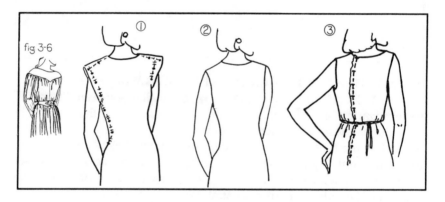

fig 3-6

Bodice Have your friend smooth the dress(es) over your shoulders. The necklines are unimportant and need not match. **4.** Match the center backs, if possible and pin together. If you've already installed zipper, match centers, then pin lining out of way of slide. Carefully pin the two garments together at the bottom of the yoke near where it joins the bodice. **5.** Pin together front and back armholes below the yokes so the side seams of the upper dress are exactly on top of the side seams of the under dress. Do not attempt to match the depth -- or even the shape -- of the armholes. Later you will *change the lining* to correspond the sheer.

Put on the width belt you will wear (if any) and arrange the gathers and blousing to flatter your figure. While wearing your strapless bra, sit in your usual fashion and check to see if the top of your bra is below the seamline of the yoke as it should be. You may need a demi-bra (which gives a very fetching impression through sheer cloth). Use the pen

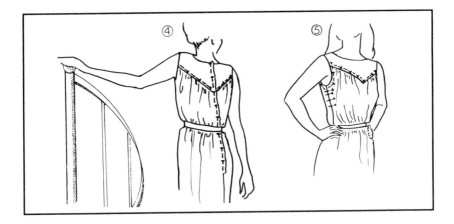

generously to mark anything you need to know, such as a notation that you need to raise the armhole of the lining pattern.

Remove the still pinned-together muslin dresses very carefully. **6.** While they are connected lay them on the table (muslin lining is underneath) on top of transfer paper, with its business side upward so the wheel marks on the lining. Arrange in such a way that the lining of the portion of the dress you are going to mark on is smooth -- you will not smooth out the bodice gathers, of course. Use big-headed pins here and there to pierce both fabrics and the cutting board to hold the two muslins together. With the wheel trace the exact location of the yoke/bodice stitchline. After marking one section, move to another. **7.** In the case of armholes (or anything else) not being as large as the outer dress, it's best to simply turn the dresses over so the lining dress is upward. Place them -- still pinned together -- on top of the lining pattern and make the correction at once, so you will know just how much you must add.

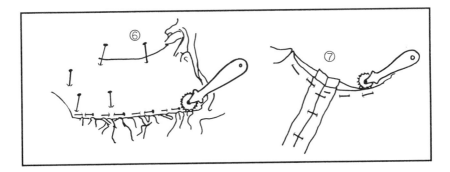

Change Facsimile Unpin to separate the dresses. Carefully rip apart the lining dress and press (no steam) the front and back. Place the lining muslin front wrong side up on transfer paper with gummy side against the facsimile. **8.** Trace the stitchline for the yoke and any armhole change not already made. Notice: you may have stretched the armholes a bit, so hold in the proper placement with pins. Trace the waistline, also, if you will belt the dress. This shows you where to sew the underskirt. **9.** Remove muslin from the facsimile and add seam allowance to yoke seam line. Cut on cutting line and discard any pattern beyond. Erase any original lines that are no longer appropriate. Repeat these steps for the back. Use # 2 to widen, if required. Use this type pattern beneath a gathered area.

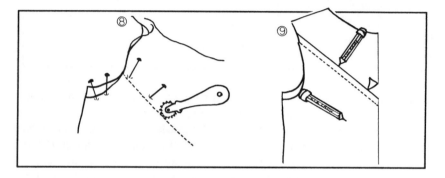

#6 UNDERSKIRT FOR GATHERED SHIFT (fig. 3-7)

Use a straight skirt pattern with one dart on each side that fits properly over your hips as a basic pattern. Determine the width of finished sheer garment at hem and jot figure in notebook. Make two facsimiles of both the front and the back.

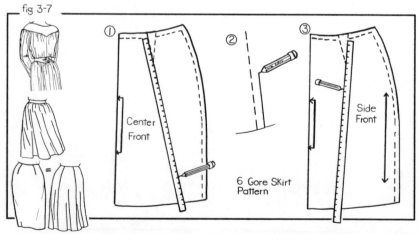

fig. 3-7

1. Lay a long straightedge alongside first leg of front dart and draw a line through the hem. **2.** Add seam allowance toward the side seam to the long line you drew and cut out. Center front is straight of grain. Label. **3.** On the other front pattern near side seam draw a line parallel to center front for straight of grain. Next, extend other leg of dart, add seam allowance toward the center front and cut out. Repeat all steps for pattern back. Center back is, in this example, not cut on fold. Follow #3 for notches.

You have a 6 gore skirt pattern which you use as an underskirt pattern. (In this case, 7 gores, because the center back is split.) Check hem measurement for size. If it's only a little too wide, narrow by #4, dividing surplus amount by 8 because you have 8 new seams to work with. Don't use side seams this time.

If dress is unfitted through waist, underskirt pattern *can* be a few inches larger than your waist measurement.

#7 WIDE PANTS GATHERED OR PLEATED TO A WAISTBAND
(fig 3-8)
Make two columns for measurements in your notebook --one for yourself and a corresponding one for the pattern. Measure your waist and add 4 in. Write figure in notebook. Put tape around your hips, sit on hard chair and note measurement. Add 2 in. and jot figure in notebook. Measure pants pattern waistband, excluding overlap, and write in notebook. Measure pattern just above the crotch and write down. Is the pants pattern still larger than your special measurements? If so, use the following method to reduce pattern slightly for lining.

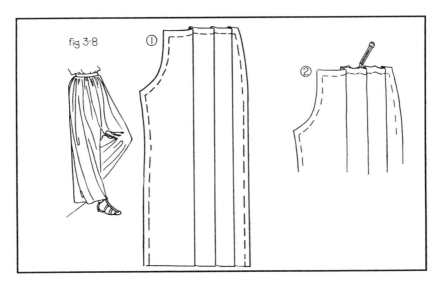

1. On the front facsimile for pants, fold out a small amount as shown. Check until the pattern measures about the size of your special measurements. You may make two or three small folds. You want the pants to be roomy and comfortable, so don't fold out too much. **2.** If

there are little points at the top at the waistband, caused by pleats in the original, snip them off and ignore. If you want more leg narrowing, use #8 below. This is your lining pattern.

#8 PANTS WITH WIDE LEGS, NO GATHERS OR PLEATS AT WAIST (fig. 3-9)

On front below crotch on inseam, narrow leg a few inches as in #4 except you curve seam in slightly just below crotch. On the outer leg seam, start narrowing below the fullest part of the hip as in #4. Add seam allowances and follow #3 for notches. Repeat for back.

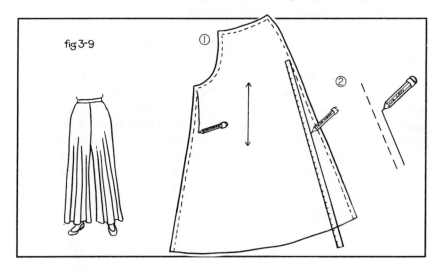

fig 3-9

#9 PANTS WITH FEW IF ANY GATHERS OR PLEATS AT WAIST, STRAIGHT LEGS (fig. 3-10)

Use the same pattern as the pants narrowing as in #8, but narrow it much less. Follow #3 for notches.

Skinny trousers are not suitable for sheers because the fabric has very little give and would rip.

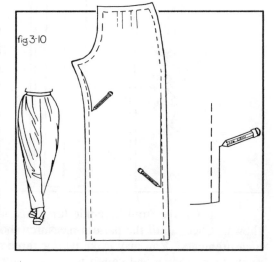

fig 3-10

#10 PANTS FULL CUT AND SEWN TO DRAWSTRING (fig. 3-11)

You can follow #7 if you are mindful that sheers cannot stretch and must be cut in the waist big enough to go over the hips with ease.

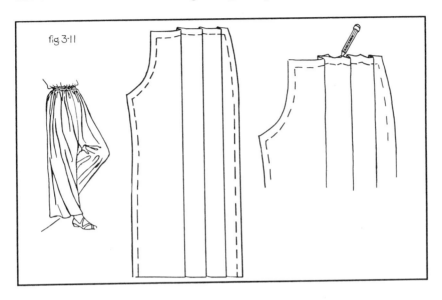

fig 3-11

#11 EXTENDED FRONT FACING CHANGE (fig. 3-12)

When the front bodice and facing are cut in one, you must add a seam for ruffle, etc. and *usually* for interfacing.

Cut 2 facsimiles of the front bodice.   **1.** On one, add seam allowance to the fold line, going into the facing area to do so. Cut on your new line and discard facing beyond. What is left is the new front bodice. **2.** On other front, add seam allowance to fold line going toward the armhole to do so. Discard the rest of the front pattern. What is left is the new facing pattern. Center fronts are straight of grain.

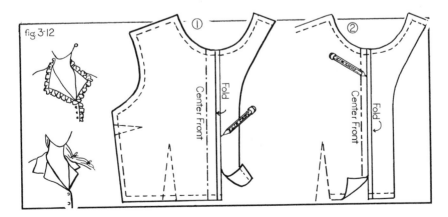

fig 3-12

#12 STRUCTURED BODICE, DARTS CHANGED TO SHOULDER FOLDS (fig. 3-13)

This alteration is for the V-neck bodice without collar or sleeves
1. On the front facsimile make a dot at the prominent point of the bust
-- usually indicated on the pattern -- and draw the underarm and waist
darts to it. Draw a line from middle of shoulder seam down to bust point.
Draw 2 more lines, one on either side of the first. **2.** Cut on the middle
line down to bust point. Crease on one leg of waistline dart and fold to
meet the other leg. Repeat for underarm dart. A big opening appears on
cut line from shoulder. Slip paper under this part of bodice.

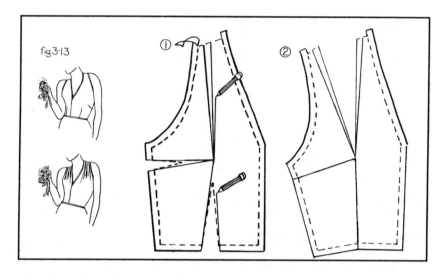

3. Cut on other two lines down to bust point and push pins in at
point to hold. Arrange space evenly. Secure all with Scotch Tape. **4.** Add
seam allowance and make little snips at outside lines to indicate first and
last tucks.

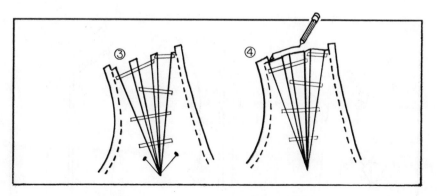

Use this pattern for top layer of the sheer, especially for chiffon. Turn the three folds toward neck and sew with shoulder seam. Baste tucks in temporarily toward bust points. Later, when you remove bastings, tucks will open as required.

#13 CHANGE PARTIAL WAISTLINE GATHERS TO DARTS IN LINING (fig. 3-14)

Unless you are quite flat in the bosom, you will need this alteration for the lining. If there is a seam holding front gathers, rip open muslin after fitting and re-pin area so you have two or so neat darts pointing toward bust point. Handle the skirt gathers the same way; point darts downward. Transfer changes to facsimile for the lining using transfer paper and the wheel similar to steps 6 and 7 in fig. 3-6. Use this for the lining pattern for the gathered area.

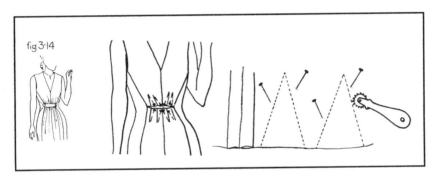

fig 3-14

#14 EIGHT GORE SKIRT FOR WIDE EMPIRE UNDERSKIRT (fig. 3-15)

Measure the front "waist," whether high or low, from side seam to side seam and put that figure in notebook. Take hip measurement all around body, add 3 in. and divide by 2; write this figure in notebook. Measure from so-called waist down to fullest part of hip and write figure in notebook. Decide the approximate length of skirt and fold a piece of drafting paper that long plus 3 or 4 in.

1. Divide waist front measurement by 8 and measure out that amount from fold near the top of paper and make a dot, A. Divide new hip figure in notebook by 8 and measure out that amount at the full hip level and mark B. Draw a dotted line connecting A to B and carry line on down to the hem. Connect bottom of line to fold. However, consider how wide you want the underskirt at the hem. If you find the proposed skirt hem will be far too wide, you have an alternative if the sheer skirt is a figured cloth, or is not sheer chiffon, or has little gathers or pleats at the top. You may increase the distance from the fold to A, even as much as 1/4 in., as shown in **2.**, which will make the hem measure less. **3.** Mark 1/4

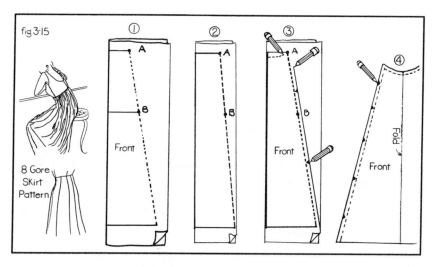

in. down at top and draw a curved line up to A. Add seam allowances to waist and sides. The length from top to bottom is the approximate underskirt length plus 3 in. Make a little snip at the fold at waist to indicate the center of the gore. Cut one more pattern just like this one if you will cut on double thickness of cloth, the usual case. Make 2 notches randomly along seam allowances. **4.** Open out *one* panel as shown and on *one* long side of it add 3 more notches.

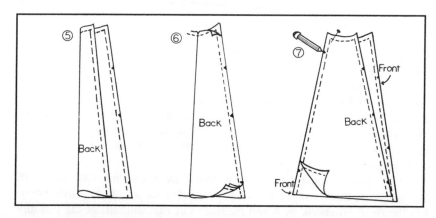

Measure back waist seam and follow all steps for the back except for notches. **5.** For back notches, put 3 random notches on one side of one panel only. **6.** Open it out and place other (still folded) pattern on top. Mark notches on seam allowances of folded pattern. **7.** Place front pattern with 5 notches on table and on top the un-notched edge of back, matching waist seams. Mark the many notches on the back and make seams the same length. These seams with 5 notches are the side seams.

Your last little job is to pay special attention to 10 in TIPS at the beginning of this chapter.

Open out all patterns for gores when you cut out. Don't bother rounding the bottoms now. When your friend marks the hem, this will be taken care of.

#15 LINING FOR DRESS WITH LOW WAISTLINE (fig. 3-16)

Depending on the garment's design and your wishes, you have several choices for lining the bodice. For the partially connected lining, cut the two exactly alike and follow the procedure in 7-2. You can use the same idea for straps over the shoulders giving the camisole look; adapt the long garment in Additional Information in the back of this book. For that, follow the general ideas in #5, 3-6, except you cut the lining for the bodice. Should you simply want a partially connected bodice lining to hang free, we give you the following ideas. A free-hanging bodice lining reaches below the flounce seam but when hemmed stops short of the bottom of the skirt. The method for cutting the flounce lining follows; flounce is always lined separately.

1. Extend the center front and side seams to the approximate length of finished dress for the lining pattern. Narrow following #4; add seam allowances. Repeat for back and then follow #3. If the waistline is only slightly lowered, check #5, and #17 and, using the most appropriate system, adjust it to your situation. Follow one of these for the bodice lining. You will have a separate lining for the flounce.

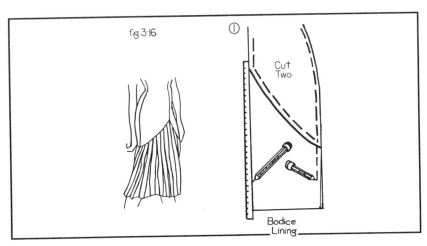

fig 3-16

①

Cut Two

Bodice Lining

2. On drafting paper draw the curve of bottom of bodice -- where it joins flounce. Extend center front and side seams on down to hem plus 3 in. Cut away on curved flounce seamline. No need for center front seam on this new pattern so make the center front stitchline the fold line.

3. Draw about 4 lines from bottom of area up to the seamline. **4.** Cut on all the new slash lines and spread 1 in. or less as appropriate. Secure with

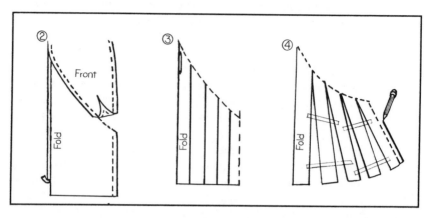

Scotch tape. Add seam allowances for side seam and flounce stitchline. Label. Repeat for back flounce pattern. Follow #3 for notches. Center front and center back are straight of grain. Cut another newsprint pattern for the front flounce only.

If you have the fabric pleated for the flounce, also make a newsprint pattern for the sheer flounce. **5.** Overlap side seams, ignoring any flare. Should there be a center front seam, disregard and put that on a fold. **6.** Pattern will be finished length and only one piece that extends from center back with a little extra for joining pleats, across front to other center back, again with a little extra for joining pleats. Arrive at correct flounce and lining lengths during the fitting of muslin trial garment.

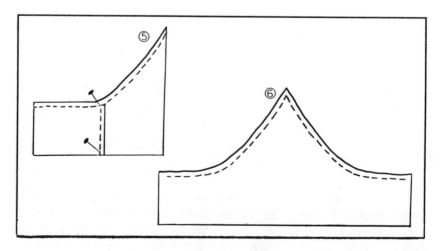

#16 LINING FOR CLOSE-FITTING BODICE (fig. 3-17)

When a fitted bodice has normally placed armholes, you can use the bodice pattern as a basis for bodice lining. (When sleeves are cut in one with the bodice, you must use the camisole.)

1. While wearing the proposed bra, put on muslin dress. Put pins where you judge to be an attractive shape across the chest and back for the bodice lining. **2.** With right side of dress upward, place transfer sheet, business side against inside of muslin dress, and trace lines with wheel. Rip top of dress apart and press with dry iron.

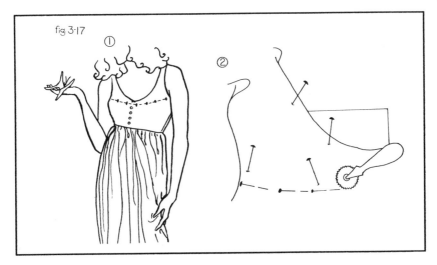

fig 3·17

3. Turn wrong side up on facsimile matching centers and edges. Hold with pins. Slip transfer paper between with its business side against the facsimile and wheel the lines. **4.** Add seam allowances to new pattern. **5.** If you want to finish the top with a fitted facing, for a pattern measure a 2-in. band to conform to the shape of the top.

Do all steps for both front and back.

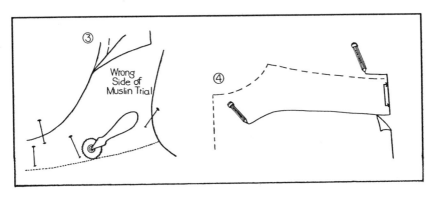

Wrong Side of Muslin Trial

Sew and test this trial lining and make any slight adjustments necessary. You will tack it at armholes and near any seams at center back or center front.

You usually wear a strapless bra, but if the outer dress is not as sheer as transparent chiffon or organza or is dark, a bra with straps the same color as your skin or one shade darker may be acceptable. Don't let the top of your bra show above the lining.

17 OPEN CAMISOLE IN BACK (fig. 3-18)

1. Add two lines beyond center back. The first is 1/4 in. beyond and it is the new fold line. The second is 1 1/4 in. from center back and you cut on this edge. From new fold to edge is facing. Adjust top facing, if any, as well.

After you sew the test camisole, alter it to fit your figure flatteringly. **2.** If back is too broad causing gathers instead of ease, fold out as needed, smooth out shape of top and reposition straps if necessary. Remember, through some sheer cloth your friends can see almost as much as if the outer garment weren't there. **3.** If your bra pushes up flesh under your arms, cut the camisole higher there and continue this addition across your back. Carry seamline up newly raised side seam. **4.** Superimpose dots as shown so additions agree. Under pattern should disappear at seam marks.

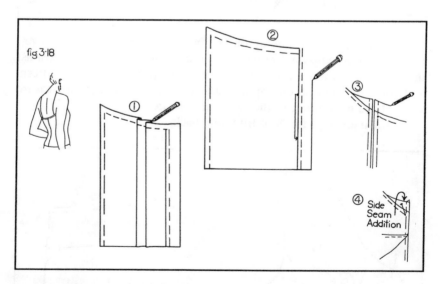

fig 3-18

Make any such changes on the facsimile following the general suggestions in fig. 3-8, illustration 2.

#18 CHANGE CUFF PATTERN (fig. 3-19)

If your pattern is sporty, you need a seam on all four sides. Add one on the edge of cuff if it's cut on the fold following the system in #11, fig. 3-15.

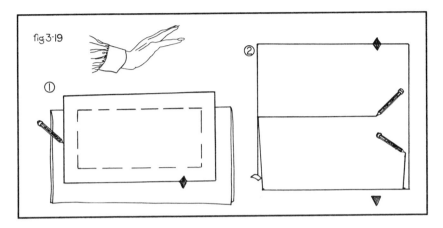

If your garment is dressy and has a two piece pattern, the kind you need for the sporty garment, you have to make a one piece pattern.

1. Fold a piece of paper and lay the bottom edge of cuff pattern on it so the seam allowance extends off the paper. Draw around the pattern. **2.** Open out and draw a line on the fold to represent the crease of cuff. Cut off notch from one side. On this un-notched edge make dots in from side edge 1/8 in. or a little less. Connect dots to edge at fold. Discard little pieces. This is the pattern for cuff and lining. For interfacing pattern, trace the half of cuff pattern from fold to notched edge.

Anytime you're faced with a lining situation, one of the forgoing systems should solve your problem.

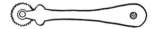

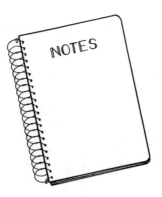

4

Let's Do Some Figuring   YARDAGE AND SHOPPING

You are almost ready for a most exciting shopping expedition. Now you have the necessary altered pattern pieces at hand and you can figure how much sheer fabric and lining to buy.

In this chapter you'll learn about a new method for figuring the yardage in order to execute a never-fail method for cutting out. The pattern layout may be different from that in the guide sheet.

Here's the way it works. You arrange pieces so they fall into natural groupings. You will cut out only one group at a time and no group may overlap another. No group should be longer than the longest pattern piece if it is a floor-length garment and the space should be as nearly filled as possible. Because commercial patterns usually give the layout for several sizes in one diagram, you may not need more fabric than indicated on the pattern envelope.

YARDAGE

Sheer Yardage

Let's assume fig. 4-1 is your proposed dress. Collect each and every pattern piece you need for the sheer fabric. You could use the following groupings: **1.** The front and one yoke. **2.** The back and one yoke. **3.** The second layer of sheer for the front. **4.** The second layer of sheer for back **5.** Sleeves and cuffs.

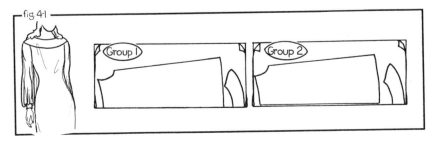

fig. 4-1

55

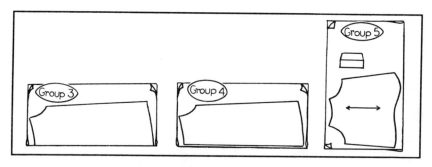

These arrangements take advantage of the fold of the cloth. However, you could also open out the cloth after the sleeve cut-out and cut the yokes alongside them and cut the cuffs near the bodice armhole. Should you want bias, you can cut it from near a bodice or sleeves, depending on the final choice of layout. Don't forget space for the belt if you will have one covered. Total the amount for the sheer and add to it about 1/2 yard for insurance and experimentation. Write the amount on your shopping list.

Lining Yardage Figure the lining similarly because it is too wiggly to manage any other way. Of course, the lining takes much less because you never line sleeves (well, almost never) and you've chosen unlined yokes. Because the street-length dress is relatively short, you can get by making only one group of the lining pieces. If you plan on a professionally made belt, experiment with belting, lining and sheer and see if the appearance is correct. Strangely enough, sometimes the belt will look like a different color and you will need to use slightly different shade for it's lining. But, if the color is correct leave space for the belt lining, too. Add up the amount of lining you need and add to the shopping list.

Of course, you have other things on your list. You may not want to buy them all at once because you don't want to make any mistakes. For instance, you don't want to buy buttons that are too heavy, or lots of thread that won't give a good stitch with your machine. Chapters 6 and 7 help you in these areas. Still, you need your shopping list complete so jot down all you need to make your garment and cross them off as you buy them. Your list may look like this:

_____ yards of sheer
_____ yards of lining
Several spools of fine thread
Fine zipper (or buttons, or hooks and eyes and snaps)
Several size 9 or 10 machine needles (60 or 70) recommended by
        your machine dealer or sewing teacher
Needles for handwork and basting
Very fine pins

Pins with big, colored heads
Soft sew-in interfacing for cuffs
Big cutting-board, cardboard or pinable
Sharp scissors, without flaw

Notice you use absolutely new pins and needles. Don't economize; one snag and your beautiful cloth is ruined. If you have to sew through paper, you will need to replace your needles more frequently requiring more needles than usual. Why the big-headed pins? They protect your fingertips and they are easy to distinguish from the other pins.

FIBERS

You will notice that sheers are located here and there in stores, not all in one place. One cloth merchant said it depends on color, kind of fiber, type garment you could make from it, price and popularity! In other words, the search is on. Look in every nook and cranny so you won't miss one bolt.

The many types of sheers force you to make a choice of fabrics while you are in the store and can actually handle and compare the various rolls. Within each category of each fiber type the hand can be different due to texture and sheerness. Always consider both in conjunction with your pattern. However, there are guidelines.

Silk

Genuine silk gives the best sensation to the skin, drapes well and looks expensive. It IS expensive. It must go to your most dependable dry cleaner. Many stores don't stock pure silk because it is so costly.

Rayon

One hundred percent rayon drapes beautifully and feels soft against the skin. It wrinkles easily and it too must go to the dry cleaners. You can often use it in conjunction with silk for some layers of underskirts if the color is correct.

Polyester

There are some fine qualities of polyester sheers on the market today and the best of these in chiffon are almost indistinguishable from silk. If you are a beginner who wants a chiffon gown or blouse, polyester is surely the answer for you. For all practical purposes, it is hand washable and you can usually dry it in your dryer. You may find that a textured weave, such as Georgette, drapes better than a completely flat weave. When flexibility and color are satisfactory and you follow the suggestions for care, you will be pleased with your polyester chiffon. If someone bumps you and spills party food on your chiffon creation, all is not ruined. Simply excuse yourself, sponge off the worst of it and go back to the party. Take care of the rest of the matter when you get home. However, organza is another matter. Silk is superior. Of course, you can't care for it the same way as a synthetic. When you have a choice of fibers such as this, always compare them so you can make an intelligent decision.

Nylon

Yes, you will find nylon sheers on the market, although it is usually hard to categorize them. It's a sheer, but what is it, you wonder. Sometimes you find such a print on a sale table for a very low price. This is certainly a good buy for a beginner; you never need to buy the most expensive when you're first starting with these procedures. Many women have made beautiful sheer garments from such fabrics. Remember, nylon cannot take as hot an iron as polyester.

LINING

Fiber

The lining must require the same care as the sheer. You can use rayon under silk because they both go to the dry cleaners. Or, rely on suggestions of your salesperson who should know about the latest fabrics available. You want synthetic lining for a synthetic garment, always keeping in mind the effect your pattern calls for. Touch and handle the linings until you find one that will enhance the design of the garment.

Color

A plain colored garment usually requires a plain colored lining. This is certainly true for the more opaque sheer such as voile. However, for a chiffon print you have lots of leeway. You want a lining color that enhances the print (and you) and one shade may make a world of difference. You will have to carry the bolt of chiffon around with you to the lining section to actually check the effect.

A word about white: a fair-skinned woman thought that since she wore a beige colored bra under her white blouse, that beige was the perfect color for cuff lining. Unfortunately, it didn't work that way and she had to throw away the cuffs. Profit from her experience: beige lining makes white cloth look dirty. For yourself always line and interface white with white. Along the same line, save those blues and pinks under white for children.

If your skin is black or very dark, wear accordingly a black, chocolate brown or medium dark brown bra under your sheer garment, keeping in mind that tricot shows less than lace through some sheers. For the lining color, choose from the suggestions above. Your dark skin showing through the unlined sleeves or yokes attractively emphasizes the sheerness of the cloth.

SHOPPING

This fabric information is pretty dry stuff compared to the sheer joy of actually shopping. As you unroll a bolt a few turns and view your hand through the web, your imagination works overtime. Such beauty! You will find a plain color with its matching lining (or that of a slightly lighter shade) easier to work with and more fashionably lasting; however, an overall print will conceal little sewing imperfections. Throughout this book you will find instructions for patterned sheers when applicable, so the choice is yours.

If you expect special help from salespeople there are several things you can do to win their co-operation. First, ask a full-time employee what time of day is the least busy, the time someone would most likely be free to help you as required. Find out if one certain day of the week is least likely to be filled with customers. If a particular salesperson is a favorite of yours, see if that person will be there when you can do this special shopping.

Make it possible for people to help you.

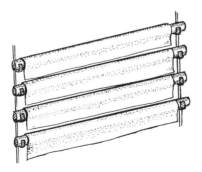

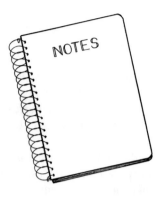

5

PREP MATERIALS AND CUT OUT

Try to allow one complete day to prepare fabric and cut out. If that is impossible, natural breaks in your work come after you prepare material, after you cut out the sheer, after you mark and label the sheer, after you press the sheer, after you cut out the lining, and after you mark and label the lining. These breaks are marked in the text by a design.

Although some of the material in this chapter pertains particularly to chiffon because of its independent nature, the general procedures are applicable to all of the fabrics. The word "chiffon" is used often, but a note is made when you need to handle another sheer differently.

PREPARATION OF MATERIAL

Silk and Rayon

Do not wet silk or rayon. Press if necessary -- check to see if steam harms the fabric -- and cut out following directions given later.

Polyester

Polyester is generally hand washable. Most pieces you can wash in the machine on the gentle cycle. You can press it with a warm iron when required, and the care after you wear it is simple. For your first chiffon garment, it's a good idea to use this practical fiber. There are some fine qualities of polyester chiffon on the market today and a beginner should consider nothing but a synthetic for her first chiffon garment. And you don't need to buy the most expensive available. When the flexibility and color are satisfactory and you follow the suggestions on these pages, you should be very pleased with the results.

When you use another sheer, buy at least part polyester with cotton so your garment will be practical and not tie you to the ironing board.

Overcast by machine the cut edges of synthetic cloth you will use in your garment, including the lining, using a sharp new needle. You will see why in a moment. Fill the washer with cool water and add gentle washing solution. Don't use regular detergent because it will make your cloth harsh and stiff. Also put in virtually everything that goes into the construction of your garment except zipper, thread and snaps.

After the machine finishes the last cycle, lift items out and re-start the machine on the final fill. Add liquid softening/anti-static solution, agitate to mix, and then return chiffon and friends to the washer to go through this last cycle again. When the machine stops this time, items are ready for the dryer which you set for permanent press. Do not add a treated sheet to the dryer because the long lengths of cloth may prevent good tumbling action and the entrapped sheet may stain the cloth.

In a few minutes the chiffon will be dry. Handling it delicately, remove it from the dryer and re-start the machine so the remaining items will continue to tumble. Go quickly to a large room and spread the fabric very rapidly full length on the floor, folding it back onto itself once if necessary. Your rush is so that wrinkles will not form while it is warm. You must use the floor because, short of a banquet hall, you will not find a table long enough to handle the yards of chiffon you require. Of course, if you make a blouse or a child's dress, a table can be long enough. Almost any other type sheer, such as voile, is not quite so delicate, demanding such speed. But still, give it your best attention.

If you don't overcast the raw edges it's impossible to unsnarl the cloth from the ravelings before a lot of wrinkles form. Always overcast raw edges.

The other items in the dryer will soon be ready to take out. You can handle the lining the same as the sheer except that its shorter length will probably fit on a table. Place the other items smoothly on a table, also. If you use a zipper, you may toss it in the dryer and press the tape with the iron set just below cotton. Although this step isn't essential, you know how the tape will react should you wash the garment later.

PATTERN

Before you cut out there are a few little things you need to do to your pattern which help you cut and sew without problems. The first is the paper stay.

Paper Stay

You pin the paper stay to the fabric neck to preserve the shape after you cut out the garment when you remove the pattern. It doesn't matter what the configuration of the neck is, it will stretch if you don't protect it (fig. 5-1). Guard the entire neck.

If the front (or back) doesn't have a seam, the facing, if any, will be cut on the fold. **1.** Fold a piece of newsprint and put the half facing

pattern on it and cut around it. **2.** Or, if the pattern has a little different
requirement, draw around the neck of the pattern making a stay about 2

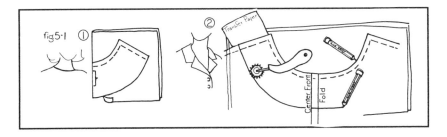

in. deep. Work on a double layer of paper if there is a seam so you will
protect both halves of the garment.

In many cases, you will also use these stays when you stay-stitch
the neck just before sewing it. Chapter 7 has more detailed information
about protection for round and V- neck. Should your pattern call for a
stay for another part of the garment, prepare it and use as you will the
neck stay.

Collar Pattern

Does your chiffon garment have a collar? To accurately preserve
its shape on diagonals and curves -- and almost all collars have one or the
other -- you need a full collar pattern cut from paper. For the standard
zigzag machine, newsprint is satisfactory -- but not newspaper with its
printing, of course, which could come off on the cloth. You can find the
right type at your newspaper print shop where you buy an end-of-roll,
which has the advantage of tearing away easily. The sensitive computerized machine, however, automatically adjusts to the thickness of whatever
it sews over. With it, when the time comes, use Solvy on top of cloth, pin
to right and left and stitch very slowly. One trick in working with chiffon
is to put yourself in the position that you need think of only one thing at
a time. Your job stitching a collar is to sew accurately without ripples.
This paper method allows that for the standard machine.

Although a sheer with more body, such as organza or voile, can
usually do without paper for stitching, every collar pattern must be full
size, not cut on the fold.

1. Fold a piece of newsprint and pin with the center
back of the collar pattern against the fold; cut around it (fig. 5-2). (If you
already have a full collar pattern, cut around it in newsprint.)   On
seamline mark shoulder seam dots, if any, centers and other signals. Mark
the grainline on the *reverse* side of paper.

Using a black felt-tipped pen draw a line on a piece of newsprint.
The Flair works well but don't get steam or water on marks -- with care
you won't. The Rub-a-Dub Sanford is waterproof but makes a broader

line. On top of the pen mark, place two layers of your sheer and one of interfacing, if you plan to use any in your collar. Can you see the pen mark well through the cloth? If so, proceed with the next step.

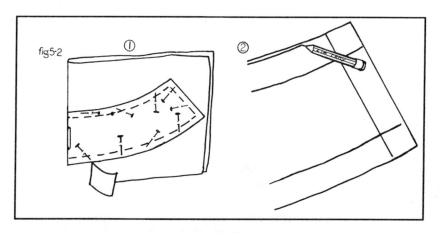

2. Mark the seamline exactly, crossing lines at corner, if any. (If you plan topstitching on a more casual sheer, one that has points, see the information that follows these instructions.) At neck draw a line starting at nothing, about 1/4 in. from end of collar, and gradually increasing to 1/16 in. and diminishing to nothing at the other end. This is optional, but helps the collar lie correctly.

The interfacing pattern has the same outside shape but has no marks. Cut a duplicate.

Guidelines for Corner Topstitching (fig. 5-3)

This little drill tells you exactly where to trim collar points so you can turn corners cleanly with no bunching of cloth to mar topstitching.

1. Lay drafting paper on the corner area of the commercial pattern and trace the seamlines as well as sewing lines. Ink the sewing lines and cut out on cutting lines. 2. Starting at collar point of drafting paper pattern, fold collar so sewing lines are superimposed. Crease. 3. Open out and ink the fold line.

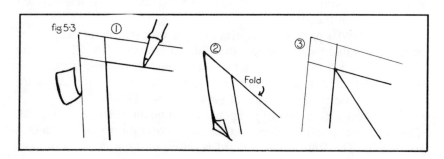

4. Again, starting at point of collar, fold so one sewing line is superimposed on inked fold line; crease paper. Through the thin paper, you can see other sewing line as it approaches point of collar. Trace this line and ink it. Open out pattern. **5.** Refold on first crease, the one in 2 and 3. Turn the paper over so the seam allowance that was underneath is now on top. Through the paper you can see the last inked line. Ink it on this side. Open out paper and cut on upper edge of this more or less diagonal line. This is the guide for the trimming line when you plan topstitching on the outside of a collar with points. **6.** Ink these corner lines on the newsprint pattern. Use this inked newsprint pattern instead of the one in the pattern envelope.

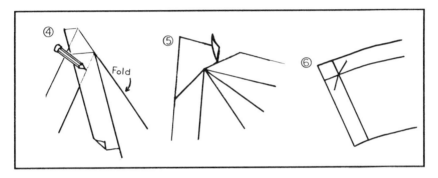

Special Connecting Dots

Although you may have already taken care of this chore, it's worth mentioning again. Prepare the patterns for tailor's tacks. If you want to take advantage of the disappearing marker, test it on your fabric fully before you use it. One you may find satisfactory is the double-faced purple colored transfer sheet which you use with the marking wheel. Although the marks don't stay on very long, it may give you time to mark later in a different way. Where are these connection dots? They're usually on a stitchline, such as where the armhole touches a wide yoke when the yoke extends over the shoulder (fig. 5-4). Fold the yoke pattern to a point at the dot and snip off a tiny bit to make a hole. You may also snip the bodice pattern seamline dot; then you know you must match these two spots. No wondering later just where to join.

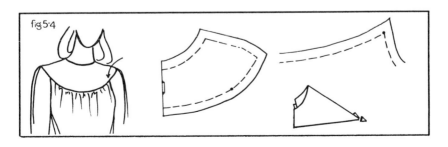

fig 5·4

Alike Pattern Pieces

Use methods that help you in meticulous work. One is to cut duplicate patterns as required, such as for the many-gored skirt, so practical in a delicate fabric. Suppose you have four gores in front and four in back. Moving two pattern pieces from place to place for the cut-out would result in trouble at the cutting-board and misshapen pieces to sew. You need only two front-gore patterns cut full-size and two for the back because you will be cutting on double fabric. Cut a duplicate of each pattern piece if they are already full-size (fig. 5-5) or use the method in fig. 5-2 if on a fold.

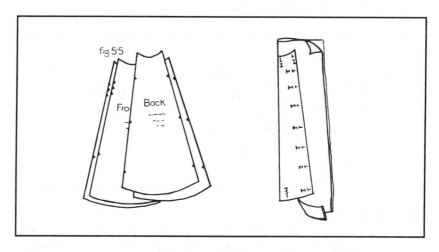

fig 5·5

Zipper

If you will use a standard zipper, make that seam 1 in. instead of 5/8 in. Add 3/8 in. to your pattern. Cut the regular 5/8 in. seam for the Invisible zipper.

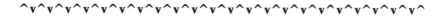

HOW TO CUT OUT

If you used a commercial pattern designed for a sheer, fitted your pattern correctly and arranged your pattern pieces in groups as suggested in ch. 4, you are probably ready to cut out after reading these next paragraphs. If, however, you are using a pattern for regular cloth and want more understanding about your type garment and the appropriate sewing techniques, the headings and sketches in the following chapters help you identify such information easily. (So does the index.) When you feel that you are fully informed, return to this chapter and cut out.

The Cutting-Board

This special method for cutting out chiffon and other drifting fabrics requires a cutting-board. The first one under discussion is the cardboard affair marked off in squares and diagonals and available at your fabric store. It measures 72 in. X 40 in. and although it folds up to 12 in. X 40 in., if you can keep it out flat -- under the bed, behind the drapes, etc. -- it will be of much more use to you. It takes a little while for those folds to disappear and there's nothing like a really flat surface to cut on.

There is also the special cutting-board you use with the rotary cutter -- in fact, there are several kinds. The rotary cutter can be a big time saver on long straight seams, and on curves, too, if you are especially careful and skillful. Most people don't have one in the very large size, so we'll come back to it just a little later.

Ready the Cloth

If the clerk tore the cloth when you bought it, trim the little whiskers and it's ready. If the clerk cut it, pull a thread from the lowest point and cut on the pulled thread-line. Unless there is a design on the fabric, there probably isn't much difference between right and wrong sides. Nevertheless, fold to the inside what you judge to be the right side. Align the two selvages and, starting at one end of the cutting-board, place them on the near lengthwise line and the evened end on a cross-line.

Beginning at the corner, push in a new colored-headed pin every 1 1/2 in. to 2 in. Make sure the selvages are exactly on the cutting board's length-wise line. To prevent the cloth from riding up the pins, put each one in at a different angle from its neighbor. Don't stretch the fabric but neither do you let a bubble form. Proceed until you have pinned enough selvage to accommodate your first group.

Next, align and pin the freshly evened cross-grain on the end line of the board, not stretching but patting and smoothing completely. When you have finished it will look something like fig. 5-6.

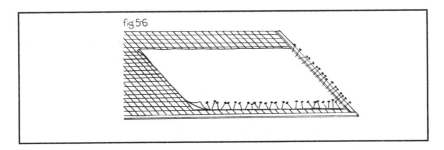

fig 5-6

Pin On Pattern

Pat chiffon gently toward the fold until it lies smoothly. Pin on the first group paying close attention to the straight of grain and which pieces need the fold. If the fabric is a little stiff, gently press the palm of one hand on the fold to hold flat while you place and pin pattern on the fold with your other hand. Does your pattern have a collar? If so, pin the new pattern with the grainline mark upward; that means the seam marks are downward. The sheer, unsupported chiffon collar goes lengthwise. Place pins as close together as you need to cut with great accuracy. Years ago many a schoolgirl rebelled when the sewing teacher made her put pins in perpendicular to the cloth. All the little girls *knew* pins should go with the seamline. Of course, the teacher was right. If you don't already do this, give it a try. Also, pin curved seams closely (and cut with the tips of your scissors).

After you have pinned on all pieces of the first group, start cutting out pieces farthest away from pinned selvages and work toward the big-headed pins. In other words, you start cutting from the fold. You don't want to remove your anchor, a very important point to remember. If you are right handed, try to cut with the pattern on your right. If you are left handed and use special scissors, cut with the pattern on your left, when possible. Have perfectly sharp scissors without flaw.

As you cut out each piece, lay it aside smoothly without folding and with the pattern still attached.

After you finish cutting out the first group (which can be only one large piece) remove all the big-headed pins and pull another crosswise thread to even. Of course, if you bought enough extra chiffon to tear each time -- no one can tell you how much that will take and you will have to be the judge -- then tear, by all means. It certainly is faster. Proceed to align selvages and cross-grain against the cutting-board lines and secure with pins as before. Pin on fresh pattern pieces and cut out the next group. Proceed in this fashion until you have cut out all the chiffon pieces.

Do not throw away your scraps because you need them to test the machine stitch and experiment with sewing procedures.

It doesn't matter what horror stories you've heard about cutting out chiffon or what defeats you've had in the past. Forget them. This method works and it works every time. It takes time but it isn't hard. Yes, you buy a bit more material but it is surprising how naturally the cutting groups form and how little extra cloth you require. Straight of grain is vital to the satisfactory performance of any garment and it is no less so for chiffon or any other sheer. By having near perfect alignment of threads down the length and across, you can hardly go wrong. The result is a garment that falls exactly as you hoped and retains its shape.

v^v^v^v^v^v^v^v^v^v^v^v^v^v^v^v^v^v^v^v

Rotary Wheel and Special Mat

With care you can slip a large cutting mat under the chiffon with its pinned-on pieces, rearrange the cloth as required to reposition it correctly and cut with the rotary cutting wheel. The small mat is all right when you use it under the first part of a group. But when you try to move it on down to finish the job, you will disturb the carefully pinned pieces. If the small mat is more trouble than it's worth, don't use it. For cutting out chiffon the large Pinable mat has the potential to save lots of time because, after you pin cloth to the mat and then pattern pieces to cloth just as with the cardboard affair, you can also cut out certain places with the wheel should you choose. But the big-headed pins must be fine and sharp and short-shanked, not long like quilting pins.

Don't use the cutting mat and wheel at the expense of accuracy.

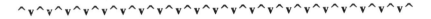

AFTER THE CUT-OUT

Marking

Check each chiffon piece to see if you indicated the notches. Also, make a little snip to form a V on the folds to mark centers, such as the center front. You must forego the old-fashioned gummy tracing paper and the wheel and substitute tailor's tacks or a disappearing marker. Using any color contrasting thread except red, hand-sew a row of stitches down the center front and center back of the garment unless they have center seams. It's a bother to try to replace the pattern on the cloth after you've removed it, so examine each piece now for omissions.

Neck

Taking great care not to stretch the neck, carefully remove the pattern from this portion of the garment and open out the cloth so the right side is upward. Slip the paper neck patterns you prepared previously beneath the sheer. After matching the cloth edges of fronts and backs exactly to paper patterns, pin and then baste cloth and paper together by hand. Using the following directions, label these pieces before you move on.

Label Each Piece

Prepare a label for each piece (fig. 5-7) so you can tell at a glance which piece is which and which is the right side. For instance, if you have an 8-gore skirt (four pattern pieces pinned to the cloth) make 8 labels, one for each and every gore in the skirt. Carefully remove one piece of pattern but don't separate the cloth pieces. Gently lift a corner and pin a folded paper label on the right side near the hem, going through only one thickness of cloth. Repeat on its mate, again on the right side. You will notice the head of the pin is near the open end of the paper label and the point is between the two layers of paper where it cannot snag a delicate fabric. Repeat for each piece.

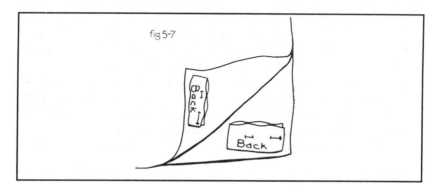

fig 5-7

If you follow the instructions you cannot make such common errors as sewing two left sleeves. Overcast the bottoms of all skirts (legs of trousers) by hand or machine. Overcast raw edges of waists by hand. Always handle cut-out pieces gently.

^v^v^v^v^v^v^v^v^v^v^v^v^v^v^v^v^v^v^v^v^v^v^v^

PRESSING

Separate one piece of chiffon from its twin and examine it carefully to see if it needs pressing. If so, take extra care that your iron is set at the proper temperature by testing on a scrap of the fabric. Almost everyone can tell a tale of woe about melting the synthetic fiber (usually nylon) of a precious dress just before an important occasion. So be sure your iron has attained the full heat for its setting before you test. Jot the setting in your sewing notebook as a reminder if necessary. Don't press over a label. When the piece of chiffon is large, push your ironing board against a table which can support the weight of the portion of the cloth you aren't pressing.

Sometimes you will buy a piece of polyester chiffon as a remnant or the end of the bolt which is so badly creased that dry pressing won't remove the creases completely. (This usually happens when the color is too beautiful to pass up or it is exactly the shade you need.) Try this: test one little portion using one of the following methods before you cut out. If you are successful, press with a dry iron as well as you can before you prepare the materials. After you have labeled the piece, you will do the serious pressing.

Place a damp press cloth over wrinkled area and press. If that doesn't work, wring out a cloth in a solution of 1/2 water and 1/2 white vinegar and press. Should neither of these methods work, throw the cloth away and don't sew with it. It will *never* look pressed.

When you interrupt the construction of a chiffon garment, lay it on a large flat surface to prevent mussing. With such careful handling you won't have much pressing to do at the finish, if any.

Special sewing procedures usually include their own pressing instructions. Often you don't press at all in order to preserve the fluid look of a sheer.

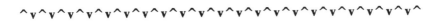

LINING

You may cut the lining following the same procedure because it, too, is slithery and difficult to cut on the straight of grain by any other method. If you don't cut the lining properly, it will poke out beneath the skirt no matter what you do.

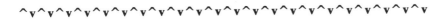

MARK AND LABEL LINING

If the lining is navy blue, black, dark brown, dark purple and the like, you may mark on the wrong side with white tracing paper and the wheel. If it is light colored, use tailors tacks or temporary marker. Mark and label each piece as you did the sheer.

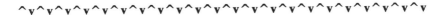

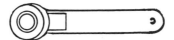

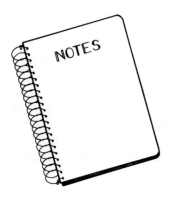

6

THE STITCH, SEAMS, FINISHES

In years past our mothers, grandmothers and great-grandmothers sewed successfully on sheer cloth at home. Did they have computerized machines? No. Did they have zigzag machines? Maybe, depending on the year. But earlier this century there was no such thing. The trusty old treadle with its woman-powered belt-driven mechanism was the sewing machine. The operator knew all the tricks in order to sew on this old-fashioned apparatus to turn out whatever clothes she wanted. She knew where to put the tiny spout of the oil can to lubricate all the moving parts and the man of the house could change the belt when it stretched too much to work properly.

If you have just learned to sew on a wonderful computerized machine, you may marvel that the woman of the past bothered to sew at all. Except for a very few sensible precautions, your machine is almost maintenance free. The zigzag isn't too far behind what with cleaning and a bit of oiling.

But those old machines could sew and that was the important thing.

No matter what kind of sewing machine you have, if it is in good repair you can sew sheer cloth with it. You may have to do a little of this, a little of that, but it will produce the stitch you need. The computerized machine probably will perform perfectly the first time you attempt sewing a sheer. Your zigzag machine may, too. If your computerized machine lacks a perfect stitch, try Solvy on top of the cloth. If there's still a problem and the instruction book doesn't help, take your machine along with some of your sheer cloth to your qualified dealer and let him help you. This step is rare.

THE STITCH

The quality of the machine stitch is vitally important to the overall appearance of your sheer garment. Rippled and puckered seams look amateurish; too long a stitch allows the seams to pull or ravel out. Spend as much time as you need working with your machine and the scraps of your cut-out garment to perfect the stitch so your finished garment will look professional.

Try the Stitch

Use either size 9 or 10 machine needle (European sizes 60 or 70) and change often if it proves you need to stitch over paper. Use the correct bobbin for your machine. Press stitching flat and then press open if applicable.

Try stitching on two pieces of your sheer. Practice making the regular stitch with 22 to 24 stitches per in. and 12 stitches per in. If the stitch doesn't look right, or if it does unpleasant things to the cloth, experiment with some of the ideas that follow.

Should your sewing machine have two sole plates -- one with a wide hole for zigzag stitches and one little round hole for regular stitches -- put on the one with the small hole. It's hard to remember to change plates later when you want to zigzag (and if you don't you'll break a lot of needles) but it keeps a soft sheer like chiffon out of the mechanism.

Place a scrap of the folded sheer on a strip of paper. (More about paper later.) This not only enables you to sew a smoother seam but it protects the soft sheers such as chiffon if you don't have the second plate. Stitch slowly. Examine the stitch on both right and wrong sides. The appearance should not be loose or tight. Tear away the paper and examine again. The fabric should not pucker. Press and re-examine.

If you are satisfied with the appearance, baste together two very long pieces of the sheer cloth that are straight of grain and re-test the stitch, again over paper. Are you pleased? Believe it or not, the long straight-of-grain seam may give you the most trouble in polyester. The center back and the center front are usually this type. You may find it helpful to grasp the chiffon (only) in your fingers behind and in front of the presser foot and hold it taut as you stitch slowly along. Be careful not to interfere with the actual feed of the cloth. This takes a bit of practice, but don't worry -- you won't have too many seams like this. If all the other practice procedures seem to work satisfactorily, just leave this problem until last and then try the forgoing method.

Next, try a long piece of bias or a piece that is at least off-grain. (This is why you save all your scraps. Pieces of other cloth won't do.)

If you aren't satisfied with what the stitch does to your sheer, read on.

Adjust the Stitch

There are five possible adjustments you can make. Three are on your sewing machine and are explained in your sewing machine instruction manual.

1. The pressure may need to be lighter or heavier.
2. The upper tension may need to be tighter or looser.
3. The bobbin tension may need to be changed.

Many "experts" say don't fool with the bobbin tension, but if you've been sewing with heavy wool how can the same setting be suitable for a sheer? The instruction manual will tell you how to make this adjustment. Do not be afraid of your machine. Remember, if you can't get the setting right and get it so messed up it won't work for your cloth, *then* you can take it into the repair shop. (Be sure to take some samples of your sheer cloth and insist the repairman demonstrates it's performance on those very pieces of cloth.) However, try all the other adjustments first.

The remaining changes are:

4. Try different kinds of thread. The choice for many women sewing with delicate cloth is either J & P Coats mercerized cotton covered, or Mettler cotton mercerized embroidery, because their fineness gives a good stitch and the sheer cloth looks smooth beside the stitches. But try all kinds if it comes to that -- nylon, silk or whatever -- and try different brands. This is quite worthwhile and you may be surprised at the difference it can make. If you are unsure about this item, hold off buying all the thread for the garment until you have a chance to test several types and brands at home after you have cut out the sheer and have the scraps to work with. If all else fails, try one type of thread for the bobbin and another type above, but make sure your machine will operate that way. Some older models require the same thread both places.

5. Change the paper you stitch over (or use Solvy). Some that have been used successfully are thin drafting paper, typing paper and newsprint, mentioned in earlier chapters. (Tissue paper is too soft.) Whatever type paper that works for you is fine. Use it when you stitch over only two layers of sheer and otherwise as required. Rather short strips of paper about 4 in. long are the easiest to handle. Simply cut a bunch about that long and about 1 in. wide and have them ready near your right hand by the sewing machine. When you stitch over the strips, arrange so the sheer extends to the right slightly beyond so you can see the seam-guide to make an accurate seam width. Touch the cloth with your fingertips to hold it on the paper strip and to guide it.

WARNING! Never change more than one variable at a time. You will have no idea what worked and what didn't.

Long Seams Cut Off-grain

Many skirt seams are not straight of grain. As you stitch along and near the end of one paper strip, slip another one in place overlapping the previous one. Do not lift the presser foot. At times you may find it necessary to *very* gently stretch the cloth the slightest amount. This helps to prevent the puckered look. But you must take care not to stretch too much or the seam will have that wavy, rippled appearance. Yes, it's a fine line but with a little practice, you will find it's not hard.

This stitch-testing business, like the muslin trial, is of vital importance. If you fail at this, your following work is wasted because puckered, drawn seams signal the work of an amateur. You will develop little tricks of your own as you sew on your sheer garment. Whatever you do that works well for you is correct.

Basting

The only reason one ever bastes is to prevent troubles from forming as you stitch. Few young women have ever basted and can't imagine doing so. However, if silk is the fiber of your cloth you may well want to baste to save yourself grief later. After all, it really takes very little time to hand-baste a long skirt seam if you lay it on a table, pin a few places and take medium hand stitches very near where you plan to stitch. If you don't baste long seams, they can drag a bit, one more pitfall to make your garment look homemade. You haven't come this far for that. Short seams, such as shoulder seams, may not need basting. Experiment with your scraps to find out.

Many a woman has more than one sewing machine. Usually, she simply didn't want to trade in a dependable old friend when she bought the newer model. If you're the lucky owner of a second machine, it's time to dust it off, check it out and put it through its paces. Almost every machine excels at one procedure, such as stitching over many layers of cloth. Should you have an underskirt, you will have some areas that have two layers of lining, one layer of underskirt sheer and two layers of dress sheer. These add up to a certain amount of bulk in spite of the relative fineness of the fabrics. This is an example of one place the second machine can be very useful -- set for this heavier stitching. Keep this machine set up, threaded and ready to go. Turn to it when it's time for its specialty.

The next logical step is at hand. You can practice your stitching skills as you try out the seam finishes.

SEAMS AND FINISHES

All seams and finishes are a matter of common sense. If you gather a piece to a sheer area, you must finish the resulting raw edge in some way to prevent unsightly whiskers showing through the sheer part, and to prevent raveling to the point of actually ripping apart. In some situations you have a choice of finishes and it depends on several things: the type seam, the sheerness of your cloth, whether the cloth is patterned or plain and the type of garment it is. For example, the skirt length and the social affair play a part in the type hem you use. In short, it's always a matter of matching the finish to the situation.

Although sheer fabric gives the appearance of utter fragility, it must be able to withstand normal wear for its design. Happily, the techniques that make the garment fragile looking also make it strong. For instance, the covering of bias binding over the sleeve/sheer yoke seam necessitates two additional stitchings, one by machine and the other by hand. This slim line of heavier cloth which emphasizes the sheerness of the fabric also gives it needed strength.

Use Your Scraps

As you experiment with these seams and finishes have your notebook handy. Simply pin samples to a page and write nearby the sewing machine settings you used such as stitch length, needle position, width of zigzag stitch and all the other pertinent information, so you won't have to figure it all out again. If you're working with a favorite pattern, jot down where you think you'll use a certain finish and then see if it proves satisfactory. After sewing the garment you can make further notations; you'll know next time.

Stitch Length

Most seams require the very fine stitch, 22 to 24 stitches per in. unless otherwise noted. To check this stitch about 2 in. and make pencil marks every 1/2 in. Count the stitches for each 1/2 in. space; adjust the machine until you average out the required 22 to 24 stitches per in. Write the information near your samples so you won't wonder next time if your settings are correct.

Topstitching, which is ornamental, uses about 12 stitches per in. This is a matter of taste, but don't use a stitch much longer or your garment will look cheap.

At times you will make regular seams and for those you use 10 to 12 stitches per in.

Machine overcasting requires about 10 zigzag points on each side per in., with a swing of about 3/16 in.

When you need to machine baste, set your machine to stitch 5 or 6 stitches per in.

Unless otherwise noted in the text, use these suggested stitch lengths.

#1 FRENCH SEAM (fig. 6-1)

Seam finishes may come and go but the one with staying power is the French seam. And why not -- it's fast, strong and easy. It's almost always used for the sheer shoulder seam, side seams of the bodice and often the long skirt seam. It's biggest limitation is that it isn't good for the greatly curved seam, such as the armhole. But there are other answers for that.

Place the wrong sides of the sheer together. If your pattern has the standard 5/8 in. seam allowance, take a 1/2 in. seam the first time, using the very fine stitch. The seam can be a little wider, but this produces the desired fine line of color. **1.** Trim to 1/8 in. from stitches. Place on ironing board as stitched and press flat, called a sandwich press. Open out, seam upward. Every seam has a direction it wants to lie. Press this seam the direction it is inclined to go; don't force it to lie the other direction. (For a deeper French seam you would normally press this seam open, but on a very narrow seam such as this, that is virtually impossible.) **2.** Lay the right sides of cloth together, folding exactly on seamline, and pin or baste. Regardless of the final seam width you choose, the final stitching must fall on the pattern's seamline; otherwise, the piece won't fit the area it joins. Again, press the seam the direction it wants to go unless there's a good reason for doing otherwise.

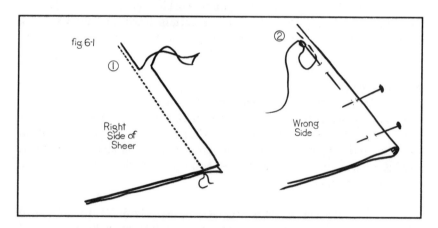

fig 6-1

① Right Side of Sheer

② Wrong Side

Because you can't trim little whiskers protruding to the right side from this seam, don't remove excess seam allowance after the first stitchline until immediately before you stitch the second time. Therefore, sew all the skirt seams the first time, set aside and then press and trim when ready to do the final stitching.

#2 TWO ROWS OF STITCHES (fig. 6-2)

Although most people automatically think of French seams when they think of sheer sewing, there are other possibilities. The two-rows-of-stitches seam takes its place in the ranks. It's a quick alternative to binding the lower part of the armhole between notches and it creates less bulk. If the skirt fabric has a pattern, it's great for sewing the many panels in a multi-gored skirt. It usually isn't suitable for the totally sheer garment such as the separate coat, and it won't stand the wear and tear of the French seam. However, choose your locations carefully and you'll like the fast results.

Place right sides of cloth together and stitch the normal seam required. Stitch a second row 1/8 in. away in the seam allowance. Trim very close to this second row. Press flat and then press the direction it's inclined to lie.

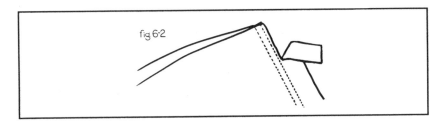

fig 6-2

#3 CLOSE ROWS OF STITCHES

This is just like the one above but the rows are *very* close together. You can use it when the resulting seam will be very visible and must, therefore, be almost decorative. Sometimes you can interchange this with the very fine zigzag.

1. Sew the first row of stitches as the pattern designates, using the very fine stitch. Make the second row of stitches 1/16 in. away from the first in the seam allowance area. **2.** Trim close to the second row but do not clip a stitch. You may coat the raw edge with clear fingernail polish. Let dry before you handle further. Fray Check is a great sealant for most things, but it is hard to control the flow for this fine work. If any gets on the body of the collar, or whatever, it will spoil it.

#4 REGULAR SEAM

Never used for unmounted sheer, the regular seam, nevertheless, has great usefulness for mounted pieces such as the mounted yoke/shoulder seams. You also use this regular seam for most of the construction of the lining. Remember to return the stitch to its normal short length if you resume sewing the sheer.

#5 OVERCASTING (fig. 6-3)

Although you may need to overcast regular seams, there's an alternative to doing it by hand to achieve that desired flat finish without bulk or stiffness. The special foot some machines have to keep the seam edge from curling as you zigzag along helps produce the flat seam required if you use fine thread and the correct length stitch. This finish means ravelings won't snarl up the zipper or otherwise cause trouble.

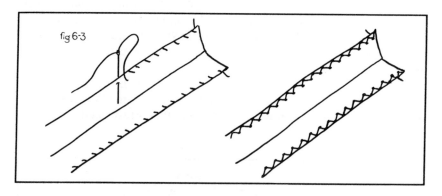

fig 6-3

#6 BIAS BINDING (fig. 6-4)

You must use this seam finish or French piping when a gathered area joins a sheer such as the bodice/yoke seam, and to bind the gathered set-in sleeve to a sheer yoke or bodice. You may use it where one ungathered sheer area joins another plain, sheer area. The general principle is also applied to finish a sheer, unadorned neck, although it is slightly different, as explained in ch. 7.

In many cases you have your choice which you will use -- this regular bias binding or French piping, which is described next. Regular bias uses less material and makes a finer finish. However, it's more trouble turning under the little edge just before the last handstitching.

Cut a strip of true bias the correct width* to produce the desired appearance. Regardless of the method, all visible seams near each other should be about the same width. Sew the seam the required amount.

1. Trim the seam allowance a little narrower than the desired finished seam width. **2.** Place one edge of bias even with the freshly trimmed edges and baste in place stretching bias very slightly. Pause occasionally, fold the bias over to the other side (as you will later sew it) to test for a smooth appearance. It should not draw diagonally. Turn over the basted piece so you can see the previous machine stitching. Stitch right next to the other machine stitching, on the side nearer the trimmed edges. **3.** Draw bias over raw edges, turn under and sew in place by hand in the seam allowance -- almost upon machine stitches. Don't go through to the right side because it will make the seam bulky and stiff. Press bias business on wrong side only.

*Figuring the correct width of bias binding is not rigid and must be arrived at by trial and error using your scraps. For the seam trimmed to 3/16 in. figure this way:

from the cut edges to the stitchline... 3/16 in.
from the stitchline to reach raw edges again........................... 3/16 in.
from raw edges on down nearly to stitchline............................ 3/16 in.
turn-under... 3/16 in.
      Mathematic total... 3/4 in.

So you cut the bias that wide, right? Wrong.

Although this figures out right mathematically, it never works out
in actuality. It's too narrow by far. To this total add at least 1/4 in. and
be prepared to add more. This variance is because you stretch the bias
before you sew, different sheers have different elasticity and the seams you
cover vary in bulkiness. Only experimentation with your fabric can tell
you what width you need.

When you test-cut bias be sure the sheer is placed carefully on the
cutting board on the straight of grain, held firmly in place with big-headed
pins and cut true bias the final width you think you need. Then place bias
strip on the ironing board and stretch it lengthwise slightly as you press
it. If this width proves too narrow, widen your next strip accordingly.
While the bias strip loses in width, it gains in length. Note the length gain
to figure the amount to cut.

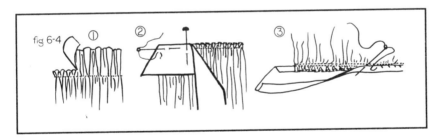

#7 FRENCH PIPING (fig. 6-5)

French piping is faster and easier than regular bias because you
are working with a pre-folded edge in the last bit of handwork. However,
it is fractionally bulkier and uses more material. In addition to the uses
for regular bias, it can be used for the upper part of the traditional cloth
placket.

Cut bias the correct width.* Crease down the center, raw edges
together. Trim seam you want to bind to measure a fraction less than you
want the finished product. **1.** Place bias, raw edges even with those of the
newly trimmed seam, and baste in place. **2.** Turn the binding over the raw
edges to the other side and carefully sew in place by hand within the seam
allowance.

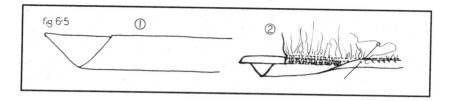

*To figure the correct width for French piping use these *general* directions:

from cut edges to stitchline .... 3/16 in.
from stitchline to cut edges .... 3/16 in.
from cut edges nearly down to stitchline .... 3/16 in.
Double this (you are working with folded cloth)............................... 5/8 in.
And because it "narrows" add to this about .... 1/2 in.
        Grand total, a little less than .... 1 3/4 in.

The measurements in this example, including the extra you may need to add, are arbitrary; use those suitable to *your* sewing situation. If your first trial proves to be the wrong width, change it as needed. Cut and handle the sheer as you do regular bias.

#8 NARROW BIAS FACING (fig. 6-6)

This is one finish you can use when applying a flat collar to a totally sheer bodice and similar situations. The finished bias width of 1/4 in. doesn't compete for the starring role, yet effectively encases the raw edges. You can also use it in place of any facing when you need a very narrow application.

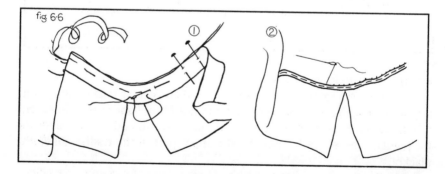

Cut bias *about* 1 1/4 in. wide. **1.** Baste the collar, ruffle or whatever, to the right side of the garment. Baste the bias in position on top. Do not try to do them both at the same time. Stitch the normal seam allowance. Trim to about 3/16 in. Clip toward seam as is necessary to facilitate turning the bias to the inside. **2.** Turn it completely to the inside so none of the bias shows on the outside. Sew to the inside of a lined area by hand going through lining only. Sew by hand or machine to a totally sheer area.

#9 DOUBLE BIAS FACING

Cut double bias just as for French piping. Use for many of the same situations as narrow bias facing. Although the single bias gives a finer appearance, double bias is easier and is satisfactory for most situations.

#10 TURNED AND STITCHED (fig. 6-7)

This is a bit of a misnomer because there are really more steps than the two indicated, but you will find it very useful. This is an optional finish for the ungathered sleeve cap, and other difficult ungathered areas when, for whatever reason, you don't want to use bias binding.

Sew the seam the regulation width. **1.** Trim the seam allowance to twice the finished width you desire. By hand overcast newly cut edges. (If you do this by machine, be sure it doesn't make the seam stiff -- something you want to avoid.) **2.** Turn toward the underside (toward the body) until the edge almost touches the stitches. Stitch to itself by hand (or machine using regular stitch) midway between the fold and overcast edge.

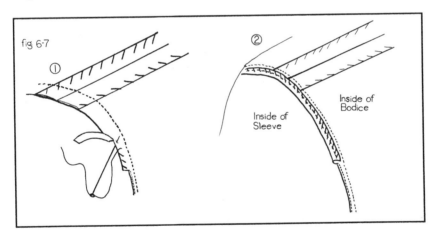

#11 VERY FINE ZIGZAG (fig. 6-8)

You use this stitch two ways but the settings are usually the same. Use the first to finish an inside area which you then trim close to the stitches. You will see this in ch. 7, patch pocket. For the second, sew the very edge of the cloth which causes the fabric to curl producing a rolled hem of sorts. This is used for the circle ruffle, ch. 9. Adjust the machine to stitch the zigzag stitch with 22 to 24 points each side per inch. These stitches have a swing of only 1/32 in. from side to side, or a tiny bit more.

1. Stitch at the location to produce the correct size. Trim very close to the stitches and coat with sealant, if desired. Often this finish is turned under and viewed through a veil of sheer cloth, fig. 7-14, step 5.

2. Stitch over the edge of cloth so the needle is barely off the cloth on the right-hand swing and pierces the cloth on the left-hand swing, causing a roll. If the appearance doesn't please you, try a wider swing.

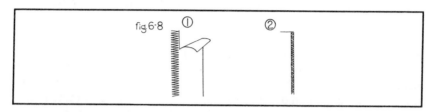

This is a perfect place to use your serger. For either serger or regular zigzag machine you may encase monofilament fishing line in the rolled hem. This produces a most professional looking edge to such things as the hem of crystal pleats well as the circle ruffle.

#12 SATIN-STITCH DOT (fig. 6-9)

Put this thread dot where you need reinforcement, especially in sheer fabric. Such a place is fig. 7-3, step 2.

Working from the right side and using fine, dull-finished thread, make a thread dot 1/16 in. round as illustrated. Rather than knot the thread, hold it on the back with your fingers and catch it in with subsequent stitches. Pack stitches close together. After you send the needle through to the wrong side completing the last stitch, send it back and forth under several stitches to fasten without going through to the right side. This little dot won't be noticeable because of its size, dull thread and placement.

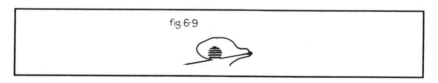

#13 BIAS-COVERED CORD (fig. 6-10)

This is an appropriate finish for armhole or unadorned neckline for a structured garment such as fig. 3-13, or at a waistline instead of a belt.

Prepare garment for facing. Cover tiny, smooth cord with bias that's wide enough to enable you to have all raw edges even in subsequent steps. **1.** Baste in position on pattern's stitchline on the right side. Then machine stitch using cording foot and regular stitch. **2.** Baste facing on top and sew in place again using cording foot but this time the very fine stitch. Turn facing to inside of garment and proceed with construction.

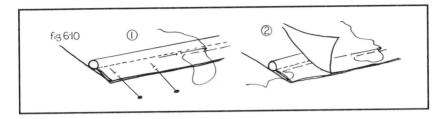

fig 6·10

#14 DEEP HEM (fig. 6-11)

Use this for such things as the top of a patch pocket and the deep hem in the skirt. The item must be straight across the finished edge like a curtain; you want no little pleats on the front or back. The deep hem can be as narrow as 1 in. for the top of a pocket to 7 in. or more for the hem in a long skirt. It's a matter or proportion and design. Sometimes you must make a judgement call. The hem in a pleated skirt **can** be as narrow as 1 1/4 in.

Here's the rule: any sheer hem that is wider than the usual narrow hem is always double. Never turn under 1/4 in. and then the deep amount. The dress will look bargain-store. (The same holds true for sheer curtains.)

1. Mark the finish line with machine basting or disappearing ink. The basting is more practical for a large area such as a big skirt. Decide on depth of hem and double it for the cutting-line. Coat edge with sealant. **2.** Fold cut edge to touch finish line. **3.** Fold on finish line and pin in place. For the deep skirt hem it is easier to handle if you baste in place.

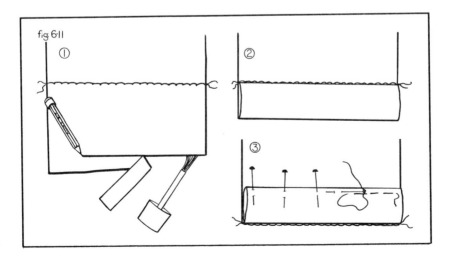

fig 6·11

4. Sew hem by machine or by hand. If by machine, (perhaps a pocket) use topstitching length. If by hand, pick up a few threads in garment with the needle. **5.** Send it through fold 3/16 in. to 1/4 in. where you bring needle out. Repeat. Remove both threads of machine basting by tugging exterior thread so it pulls the interior thread within reach.

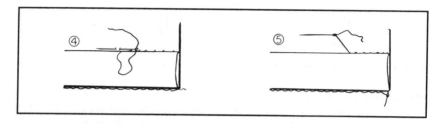

You may press the top of hem where you stitched. Press the lower edge if you like. If you're sending the sheer off to be pleated, you can baste in lower edge, too, and in between if the hem is quite deep.

#15 SIMPLE NARROW HEM (fig. 6-12)

Use this finish for the hem in the close-fitting sleeve, capes and the like where you want an unobtrusive hem. It is fast, easy and looks neat. Machine hems are in ch. 8.

1. Turn the edge to the wrong side a scant 1/8 in. and baste in place by hand with a tiny running stitch. **2.** Turn under again 1/8 in. but don't baste or pin -- just hold the turn with the fingers of your left hand as you sew in place with your right. (Reverse the process if you're left handed.) Pick up a couple of threads of the sheer and then **3.** send the needle through the fold. Stitches should be no farther apart than 1/8 in. Repeat. For a very wide skirt you can use a running stitch. Remove basting.

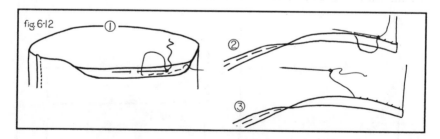

fig. 6-12

#16 ROLLED HEM (fig. 6-13)

You may use this hem for capes, wide sleeves and the like. This is the traditional hem for the chiffon skirt. However, it's hard to do and takes a lot of time. Practical machine hems are explained in ch. 8.

Run a basting thread to use as a guide. Cut about 1/8 to 3/16 in. beyond thread. Dampen your left fingers and roll the edge of sheer tightly several turns. **1.** Hold with your left thumb and forefinger while with your right hand you take a tiny stitch in sheer cloth and run it through the body of the roll diagonally for 1/8 to 3/16 in. The needle will exit the roll about half way up. Take another little stitch in the sheer about the same distance away and repeat. When finished, remove thread guide.

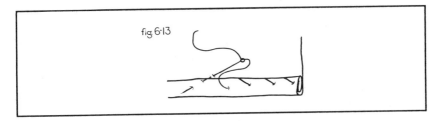

fig 6·13

#17 CONTINUOUS THREAD DART (fig. 6-14)

Although they have been in the instruction manuals for years, these next two procedures have been made popular by Margaret Islander, well-known founder of Islander School of Fashion Arts, who has helped many women sew with confidence. Her video Industrial Shortcuts For Home Sewing demonstrates the process.

If you must have certain darts this is a very neat way to handle them in a sheer area. You won't want to bother with too many because you have to re-thread the machine backward every time due to the fineness of the eye of the machine needle. However, two such darts are probably all you have. Thread must match the sheer cloth exactly.

Bring bobbin thread up and remove thread from the needle. Using bobbin thread, thread needle from the opposite direction than is usual, tie to the upper thread in a very tight square knot and pull up toward spool. If it balks at going through the tensions, thread by hand backward, wind this bobbin thread on a spool and place spool on holder.

Start at what is usually the end of the dart. Insert needle on the very edge at fold and slowly stitch toward wide top. Press the correct direction over a ham.

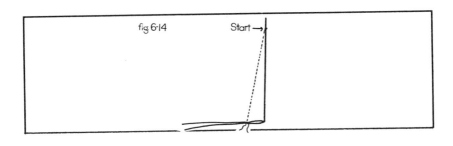

fig 6·14   Start →

#18 CONTINUOUS THREAD TUCK (fig. 6-15)

If one end of the tuck is exposed and the other is encased in a seam, start at the exposed end. If both are exposed, you have to tie threads at the finish end on the wrong side. We assume for this example that the finish end is hidden in a seam.

Place needle correctly for the starting point of the line of stitching. Lower needle into cloth on the exact spot of the first stitch and bring the bobbin thread up. Remove thread that's in the needle, send the bobbin thread through the needle's eye opposite from the usual direction and re-thread as above.

Start sewing on the spot where the thread emerges and finish at raw edge in seam allowance. Re-thread for each tuck.

If the start of the tuck is to be soft, as in the illustration, do not press the open end of it. Starting a little way from the beginning, press tuck the correct direction.

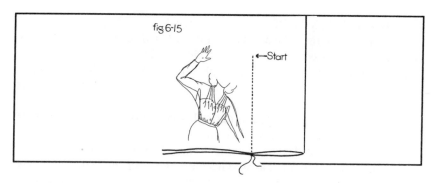

fig 6-15

←Start

#19 SEALANT

Sealant can be a valuable ally in sheer sewing. Always let it dry thoroughly before you proceed.

#20 GRADING

When many layers of a seam will be enclosed in a seam finish, such as those in the applied front blouse facing, grading can keep the turned-back edge from having a bulky ridge. After you stitch such a seam, trim each layer of cloth in the seam allowance a little different amount.

7

SEWING ABOVE THE WAIST

At first glance the routine accomplishments in regular sewing seem impossible in a sheer because everything is so visible. Many byproducts of regular sewing are hidden by opaque cloth. But, like anything else, it's all in knowing how. If you use the seams and finishes demonstrated in the preceding chapter with their practical application in these following pages, you can find your way successfully through almost any challenge of sheer sewing, including chiffon which many consider the most difficult. In this chapter we deal with sewing above the waist such as shoulder seams, neck finishes including collars, front closings and buttonholes, patch pockets, yokes and sleeves. Of course, not every single detail of sheer sewing can be covered, but you learn the principles and you apply these to similar situations.

A little reminder: be vigilant about bastings trapped between the layers even when the instructions don't warn you. It is so frustrating to see a thread you cannot reach, when it's there for all the world to see.

Experiment with the scraps from your sheer garment to perfect any technique described on these pages if you feel unsure of your skills.

#1 SEPARATE SHEER GARMENT (fig. 7-1)

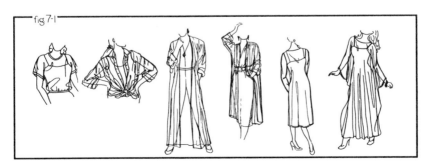

Finish every seam completely -- shoulder seams and more or less straight long seams with French seams. Finish greatly curving seams, like armholes, with bound seams. Do any required hand work to the best of your ability because you want no escaping threads to mar this chic garment. Details of collars, sleeves and other items follow.

With casual clothes you have greater latitude and may try such methods as serging, ch. 9.

#2 PARTIALLY CONNECTED LINING (fig. 7-2)

In preparation for finishing the neck, a most essential "first" step, do the following:

1. Making regular seams sew side seams of *lining* from armholes down, and center back seam below placket opening. Overcast each edge. If there's an underlayer of sheer, sew center back seams (below placket) and side seams in French seams. Repeat for the top layer of sheer, the upper garment. The three layers must agree exactly where the backs join, which is from neck to the base of placket. All zippers and plackets are covered in ch. 8 but for now, measure each layer carefully down from neck; be prepared later to pick out one or two stitches in one layer or the other. **2.** If you could open out flat on table each group would look something like illustration 2. Of course, you cannot because each one is partly joined in center back.

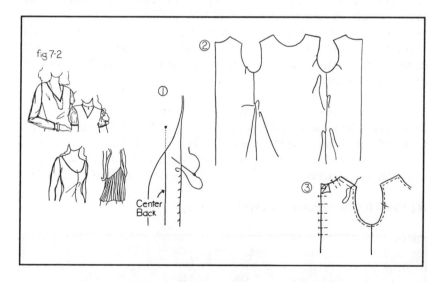

fig 7-2

Center
Back

3. Place lining on table, right side up. Remove paper stays long enough to do the following that concerns the necks and then replace one under the lining: on lining place underlayer of sheer and match at necks, shoulders, part way down center backs and armholes. (Garments with yokes join at top of bodice instead of neck.) Pin and baste together. Place top layer, the outer garment, on top. Pin and baste all three layers together. (If you're working with sheer yokes, your next step is to sew prepared bodice to sheer yoke following the pattern instructions. Bind yoke/bodice seam and then make French seams at shoulders.) Sew shift layers together at shoulders making a standard seam. Press open and overcast edges.

If your garment is a simple shift, you can proceed to face neck as with any opaque cloth, or you can bind as described for various neckline shapes below. Should your garment be sleeveless, use the same treatment for the armholes.

If your garment has a very low waistline, you may handle the bodice lining like this and then let it hang free to below the "skirt" or flounce seam; it does not reach to the skirt hem. The flounce has its own lining.

Sleeves and their installation are handled later.

FINISH THE NECK

All who sew know the neck of a garment can stretch and change shape to the point of not fitting. That's why, after sewing the shoulder seams, it is usually finished first. The idea of a round or V neck in a sheer -- especially chiffon -- keeping its shape looks impossible at first; but take your time and you will succeed. Should the garment not have a lot of weight on it, such as a plain blouse or a dress partly supported at the waist, the high round neck, even in chiffon, need no more beyond staystitching. However, the V-neck and the low round neck need help. In all cases, the goal is the same: to preserve the neck shape so mysteriously that the method is invisible. In an area of chiffon only, that becomes doubly important -- how can you manage the illusion of complete fragility?

Tape Seam tape of the non-stretch variety is your hidden assistant. There are other things you can use instead -- the appropriate type and color of ribbon or a length of selvage -- but we'll say seam tape or just tape. It is soft, comes in a wide variety of colors, is readily available and is easily trimmed. Get the type that is flat and has no design woven in its surface if you're working with a pastel.

The color you use is important. Although the same color as your chiffon is a good choice because it emphasizes the sheerness of the cloth, there are no hard and fast rules. Your skin color and the lining color are other possibilities. Duplicate the layers with scraps to decide.

If your pattern is designed for neck binding, you will follow its instructions. But if it is cut for a facing, the following paragraphs tell you what to do. Of the several bound-neck finishes that follow, all are a variation of the V-neck so read it regardless of the exact neck shape you need to bind. Notice that at some point during the course of binding the neck you will trim away the pattern's seam allowance in order to achieve the correct finished neck size.

#3 SHEER V-NECK, BOUND (fig. 7-3)

The V-neck is more or less bias and needs protection regardless of the type sheer you use.

If your garment opens in the center back, it sometimes fits in better with the construction to finish the last two inches of the neck on either side of the center after you complete the placket, whether it is a zipper or a cloth-bound opening. However, even if this is true, you still staystitch the neck to protect it. You may even put a small stay there if it is bias, such as a deep V in the low-cut back of a cocktail dress.

1. Turn bodice wrong side up. The paper stay is upward, too, and its neck edge is even with edge of the sheer. Measure from neck edge exact amount for stitchline for binding -- in this case, 5/8 in. + 1/4 in. for binding, making 1 1/8 in. in all. Mark. Send a pin through the point where these lines cross and mark spot on right side. Cut away paper stay around this spot. This is where you will pivot the machine needle.

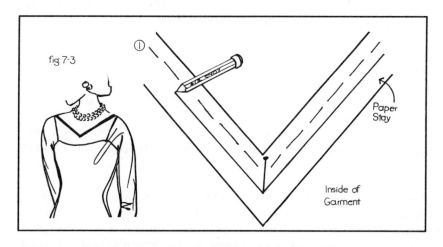

fig 7-3 · Paper Stay · Inside of Garment

2. Make satin-stitch dot on mark on the right side. See ch. 6, #12. **3.** Cut a length of seam tape a little longer than the shoulder-to-shoulder measurement and at the midway point, cut almost to 1/16 in. of edge of tape. **4.** Next, cut out a little more of a V.

5. On wrong side pin that spot at the satin stitch dot. Because V-necks are not always a straight line, you may need to clip the tape occasionally along the legs of the V so it can conform accurately to the neck shape. Pin tape to neck touching pencil line and then baste. It is

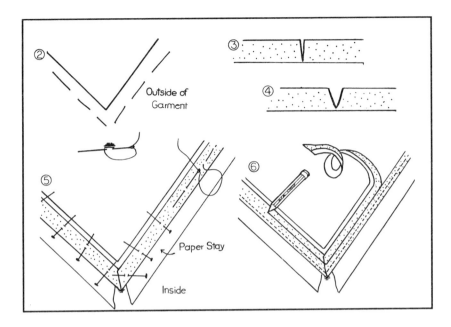

hard to make the tape come to a sharp point at the base of the V. That's the reason for the satin-stitch dot -- to protect the sheer cloth.

     6. Machine-stitch tape 1/8 in. from unclipped edge (stitchline) using the very fine stitches. Also, measure from the edge of tape toward the neck the depth of finished binding, in this case 1/4 in. Cut through all layers of cloth and paper. Remove bastings and tear away paper. Tape stops at shoulder seam unless back is also wide or low.

     7. Turn right side upward. With raw edges together, pin midpoint of bias to the satin dot. Mark pivot point on bias binding and pin bias to the neck edge for about 1 in. terminating at the dot; baste. Machine-stitch using very fine stitch for 1/2 in. and stop in dot. With needle down, pivot cloth and stitch again for 1/2 in. You may give a little snip to the bias in its seam allowance so it will adjust to the second leg of the V more easily.
8. Finish pinning and baste bias in place, raw edges even.

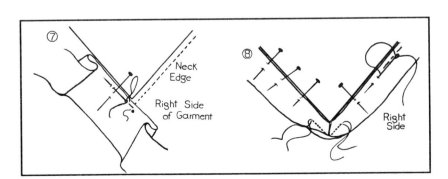

9. Turn over, wrong side of garment upward so you can see where to place machine needle, and finish stitching 1/16 in. in from the edge of seam tape. Overlap previous stitching. You are stitching on the seam tape, not on the sheer. Remove bastings. **10.** Take bias over to inside of garment. On right side with the point of your needle push in the little bubble of cloth that forms in the bias at the base of the V and hold it in place with a pin if it won't stay put on its own. Do the same on the inside. **11.** Sew bias in place in the tape area, not going through to the other layers. Sew the little fold of bias to itself on the back. The front

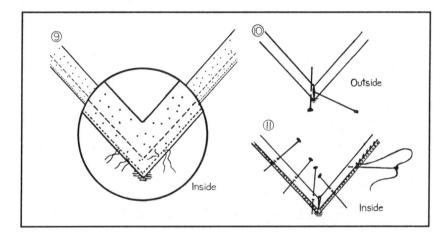

probably won't need it. If chiffon is your fabric, baste instead of pressing. Press gently if a stiffer sheer.

Only a fine line of seam tape is exposed beyond the binding. No one will ever notice the thin line if you chose the color well.

#4 SHEER WIDE OR LOW ROUND NECK, BOUND (fig. 7-4)

The strengthening of this neck shape is essentially the same as for the V-neck. **1.** To help the tape lie flat as it follows the line of the dress neck, clip it frequently along its length. **2.** Cut another facsimile of the

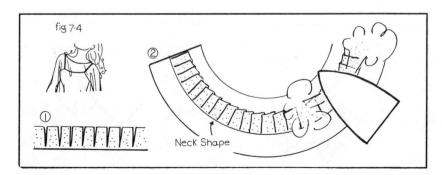

fig 7-4

round neck shape, mark stitchline for bias binding as in 7-3 and lay clipped tape along line. Steam-press tape to this general shape. If tape makes points on the woven edge instead of curving nicely, you need to make clips closer together. Proceed as for the V-neck, but there is no satin-stitch dot, of course. Notice that the sharper the curve, the more you need to stretch the bias as you baste it in place.

The finished binding will lie flat. Press as above.

YOKES

Shoulder yokes present an interesting choice -- cover your shoulders with just a delicate veil of cloth or back the veil rendering it impenetrable.

The sheer yoke takes less cloth and is a little easier. Abbreviated instructions are as follows: Sew the side seams (separately) of both bodice lining and bodice sheer. Then, as described below, gather the sheer to lining, join bodice to yoke and bind resulting seam. Join shoulder seams in a French seam, bind the neck and you're ready to move on to the sleeves.

However, mounted yokes make the garment more versatile. Incorporate that with the blouse, teaming equally well with hostess trousers, long skirt or suit, and it's the most usable of all. Sleeves are always gloriously sheer offering you contrasts in transparency. Georgette or a pebbly-weave chiffon is perfect over a very soft, silky lining. Cut yoke facing from the same lining fabric. Everything about this blouse is frankly feminine so topstitching isn't appropriate.

This is a continued story. Begin the exciting mystery of NO VISIBLE SUPPORT For the

#5 MOUNTED YOKE, Part I (fig. 7-5)

We use a familiar yoke and make a blouse.

1. Join yoke *facing* at shoulders. If there's a back shoulder dart, press it toward the arm. Clip on either side of dart to shoulder seam so dart can continue toward front; otherwise, press seam open. By hand, using a running stitch, sew shoulder seam to yoke. These permanent stitches insure perfect flatness; they are inside and won't show. Staystitch outside edge using very fine stitches, positioning them a hair more than seam width. If yoke is rounded, clip to staystitching. Baste outer edge of yoke toward wrong side by hand on staystitching. Set aside.

Mount sheer yokes to lining fabric. Staystitch a tiny bit less than the seam allowance. Clip toward staystitching only where shown. Set aside.

Join bodice lining side seams, right sides together, making regular seams. Make French seams (or other) in Georgette side seams. Put

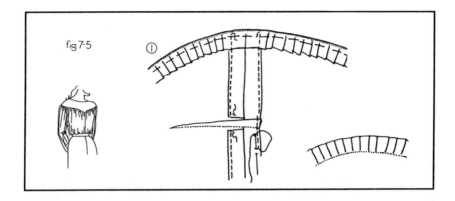

fig 7-5

gathering stitches in sheer front bodice for gathers. (If you don't know how, see CUFFS, under SLEEVES.) **2.** Draw up gathering threads to fit lining, matching centers, notches and armholes. Unless your instructions say differently, omit gathers for about an inch on either side of center front to avoid the ballooning effect. Hand-baste together at armholes and yokes, front and back. Make a satin-stitch dot at center front (and back as required) exactly where seamlines cross at base of center yoke. **3.** You may need to clip bodice a little (shown without gathers) to facilitate sewing yoke/bodice seam in that area, but don't do it yet.

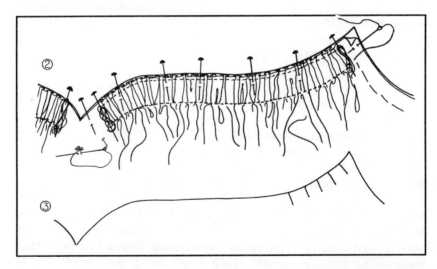

4. Place yoke on bodice, right sides together, so center front V on yoke is exactly on top of satin dot. Curve the yoke seam and baste in place as far as you can manage without having difficulty with the layers underneath -- when they will no longer allow you to stitch with ease. This is approximately the amount clipped in the sketch. Stop basting and stitch that part starting at satin dot. Fasten thread at dot.

5. Turn work over and baste as before toward armhole clipping bodice as required to allow bodice curve properly over yoke. Take care that you baste so yoke staystitching will be hidden after machine stitching. Stitch on machine, overlapping other stitches. Stop stitching at armhole seam, X. Fasten thread well. Continue in this fashion as you sew other parts of yoke, turning work as required. The reason for this back and forth business is so no topstitches rob the yoke of its softness. Baste yoke/bodice seam toward yoke. Do NOT press. Do not remove gathering threads.

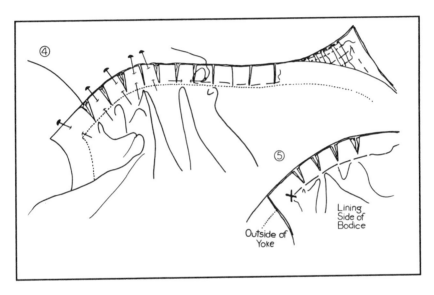

Remove enough of the neck stay to join shoulder seams in a regular seam. If there's a back shoulder dart, handle as for the facing but press it the other way to avoid bulk. Press shoulder seam open over a ham using the vinegar-water solution if necessary to do a good job. Set aside.

Read the fascinating conclusion to the mystery in SLEEVES.

#6 MOUNTED V-NECK OR SURPLICE CLOSING, EXTENDED FACING (fig. 7-6)

Although you can use the mounted system for any sheer, it's especially suitable for chiffon or Georgette. The surplice closing, with its folded-back facing and set-in sleeves, is perfect for the woman who wants something both dressy and tailored at the same time.

As these directions start, you have not yet mounted chiffon. Remove any paper stay from lining, but handle fabric carefully. The V-neck with seam at center front is used as an example.

1. Make random marks across the facsimile fold line. Cut tiny holes in the facing area, not in the bodice itself. If you have not already done so, mark fold line on inside of lining.

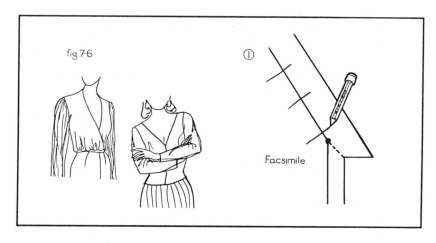

fig 7-6

① Facsimile

2. With lining wrong side up, place facsimile on it and mark dots through little holes. Mark seam tape also and indicate which end is shoulder and which base of V. The tape stops just short of base of V and does not go beyond shoulder seam. **3.** In facing area, lay tape against fold line. Sew edge that's against fold line on machine with very fine stitches. Sew other edge by hand.

On right side mount sheer layer(s) to lining. **4.** With exactly matching thread and working on the inside of lining where you can see fold line, make tiny back-stitches about 1/2 in. apart on fold line to hold all the layers together. (This will make small thread loops on the inside where you work.) You want no topstitching to do the job. Bring extra chiffon over edge of facing and sew by hand.

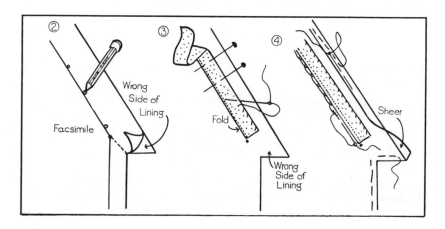

② Facsimile Wrong Side of Lining

③ Fold Wrong Side of Lining

④ Sheer

Mount the sheers for the bodice back as you did the front and proceed to follow the pattern's directions about joining the shoulder seams and back neck facing.

Surplice closing with fold-back self-facing is handled similarly.

COLLARS

The simple neck is perfect for some women, but many others like the softening effect of a collar. As with all sheer sewing, accuracy is the rule.

#7 BASIC FLAT COLLAR (fig. 7-7)

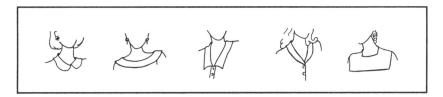

Make the flat collar dressy or casual depending on the choice of fabric and details. If you plan to toss a casual sheer in the washer, you have to do topstitching. But wash the totally sheer chiffon collar by hand. The elegance of it, soft and sheer when made in chiffon without interfacing or topstitching, is perfect for the no-nonsense woman who says she's "not the chiffon type."

Although it is unusual to see topstitching on chiffon, it does make a certain statement. Don't expect it to react to your efforts as would an ordinary fabric, however. Use another layer of chiffon if you want a bit more body. It will still have that soft look. Try voile or another more casual sheer for a conventional look. For collar stiffening, finest polyester bridal illusion in cream color is almost invisible with a light colored sheer. Some stores have such a variety of colors you can buy it to match your sheer. Organza works well, too. But test it between two layers of your fashion fabric against your arm to see how you like it.

The pointed collar is used as an example. Using heavier sheers, you can make scallops and other sharp curves but in chiffon, where you have to stitch twice, gentle curves are best. After you have followed the general instructions, try to turn. If difficult, clip several times at the difficult spots taking great care to cut through only the outside row of stitches.

Have cut-out collar with its attached newsprint pattern chiffon upward. Place any interfacing on top and pin in place. Baste all layers together, including the paper, so you can concentrate on the machine-stitching. Baste just into collar portion beyond inked seamline, which you should be able to see through the layers of cloth. If your machine is computerized, fold paper out of the way underneath and put Solvy on top.

1. Stitch on regular seamline. When you come to a collar point, if any, put needle down in the cloth and pivot collar sharply to execute a sharp turn. Continue stitching around collar slowly and accurately because this line becomes the outside edge of the collar. Next, smooth layers toward collar neck and trim wayward sheer cloth that extends beyond paper. Then, pin upper collar out of the way at the neckline and trim away the little premarked strip from undercollar. Cut through paper, too; it gives stability to the process. **2.** When there's interfacing, slip your fingers between upper and lower collars and baste the two upper layers together. They now act as a unit. **3.** If you plan topstitching, fold paper back in position, if required, and trim exactly on second marked line using the rotary cutting wheel. Seal edges as below.

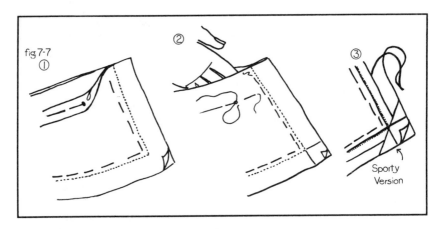

However, for the dressy collar, remove bastings and carefully tear newsprint from outside edges. **4.** Next, pin collar on newsprint again (or use Solvy) to start the second stitchline for close row of stitches. When you are almost even with the corner, put needle down, turn collar and take two stitches (or more, as required) on the diagonal to pass near the sharply turned corner. Resume stitching, treating other corner the same. Tear away paper making sure you have removed every bit of it from under stitches. Trim closely to last stitches, leaving a hairline of cloth next to them. Coat newly cut edges with sealant --delicately at the corners so it doesn't seep onto collar itself. You may find clear fingernail polish with its easy-to-manage applicator safer to handle. **5.** Turn collar. Holding upper collar toward you as you work edges with your fingers, baste close to the seam. Pin and then baste neck edges together. Overcast. Label which is upper collar.

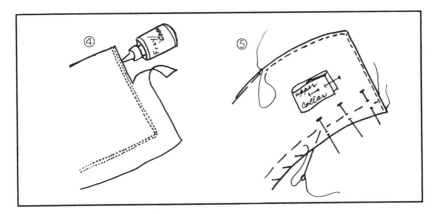

For the tailored but dressy collar, leave in bastings and you're finished. For the sporty affair, leave in bastings and press edge with vinegar-water solution. You must topstitch because you left the wider seam inside. Edgestitch (if appropriate), using a special foot with its guide if your machine provides one, and then stitch exactly 3/16 inch from the edge (or whatever you've planned) catching in seam allowance.

Do all procedures accurately because you can see all the work through the delicate web.

#8 BASIC FLAT COLLAR, MOUNTED

Mount chiffon on lining fabric this way: If the chiffon has a pattern, mount one layer of plain chiffon on lining fabric and on top put the patterned chiffon. (At least this is a starting point. You may change your mind after experimentation.) If the chiffon is a solid color -- no design -- use two layers of chiffon on lining fabric. Baste layers together and handle as one layer of cloth. No need for special sheer sewing techniques to sew the collar. The way you sew it to the back neck of the bodice depends on whether the bodice is sheer or opaque.

You seldom need to mount more opaque fabric.

#9 SHIRT COLLAR WITH COLLARBAND AND FRONT BAND
(fig. 7-8)

Not only do these appear together in a pattern, but they are handled the same way. It's unorthodox to want topstitching on chiffon but if so, here are special directions to do just that. More often you will be working with a fabric that's not quite so transparent; sometimes you can sew them according to the pattern directions.

You say you don't want topstitching? Then don't make a shirt. It's a lot of trouble requiring exacting sewing. You would be much better off making a blouse with its fold-back facing and standard collar -- no bands to worry about.

Interfacing seldom figures prominently when you sew with soft sheers because you want the fluid look. However, the shirt, by virtue of its styling, is a tailored garment and demands a little body in the collar and, perhaps, in collarband and band down the front. If there are cuffs, they need support. Standard interfacings don't bring the satisfaction they usually do in opaque cloth. Color can cause problems unless you are sewing with black or white. Fusibles often bleed through. Try one of the following suggestions.

1. Use a second layer of the sheer itself, if it has no pattern. 2. Mount layers on fine poly/cotton or lining as explained in FLAT COLLAR, MOUNTED, above. It's a lot easier in the long run, but changes the look completely. 3. Place a layer of finest tulle or bridal illusion from seam to seam on the facing. It invisibly gives the most body, as explained in the next paragraphs.

The front band for buttons is used in this demonstration. Handle the collarband similarly except you will have to trim closer and snip curves. For collar, see #7 FLAT COLLAR. Follow pattern instructions for installation of collar and collarband.

Figure 7-8, illustration 1., is one example the front band pattern for buttons. 2. Join front band to bodice front, right sides together using very fine stitches. Trim to width you want topstitching from edge usually 3/16 + 1/16 in. Coat with Fray Check and let dry. 3. Sew band facing to band, right sides together using very fine stitches. Trim like the other side and coat.

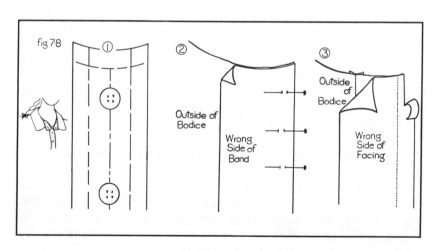

4. Press both seams toward band. 5. Pin or baste facing back to wrong side. Turn under facing seam allowance in such a way that it touches the stitches at bodice/band seam. Pin closely (or baste) and press well to crease this fold.

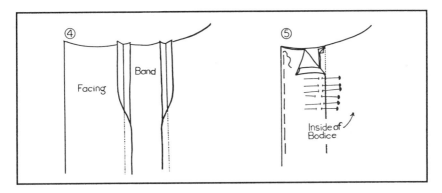

6. Open out and if crease isn't easily seen, mark with disappearing ink. Trim the correct width and coat with sealant. If you want body, cut a strip of finest tulle to fit from seam to seam and almost touching stitches. Fold facing seam allowance over tulle. 7. Lay facing back in place against band and pin and then hand-baste in place. 8. Turn to right side and topstitch about 3/16 in. back from edges.

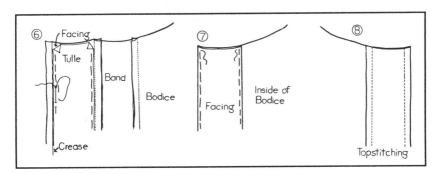

Be sure to experiment with any interfacing because it makes the sheer unexpectedly stiff.

This quiet beauty reaches the height of elegance when made totally sheer and accented with tiny rhinestone buttons.

#10 SHEER LAPEL, EXTENDED SELF-FACING (fig. 7-9)
Although this sheer tailored collar with its extended self-facing forming the lapel takes time and exactitude, it's extremely elegant when well executed. Perfect for the non-ruffle type who wants something subtly charming. There is no interfacing and no topstitching. It is described with a sheer, unmounted bodice.

1. Pin and then baste completed flat collar, right side upward, to right side of bodice at neck, raw edges even. (The under collar is against right side of bodice.) Machine-stitch, trying for 1/16 in. less than the seam proposed by the pattern. 2. Put on trial garment, turn back lapel on its

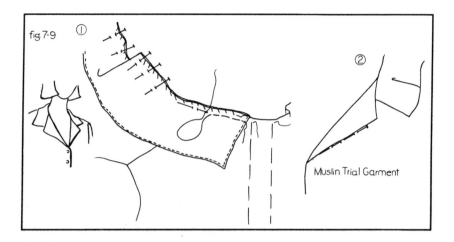

fold line, and mark along its edge with pins. Transfer pin locations to the chiffon garment.

3. Fold back self-facing and make a mark 1/4 in. above this on raw edge of facing. **4.** Open out facing. At dot clip in the seam allowance, usually 1/4 in. and coat edges of cut with sealant. Let dry. Above this point turn edge under 1/8 in. and baste and then turn under another 1/8 in. and baste. Below this clip, do the same but turn the opposite direction. Baste folds to facing only, not to bodice.

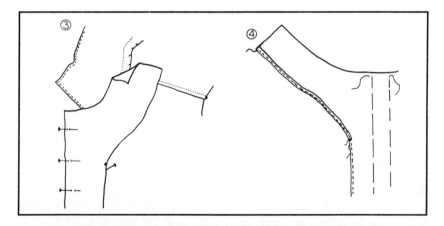

5. Turn facing to outside of bodice and baste along front fold line. (This particular basting step may seem like it's unnecessary, but you want the finished front to lie perfectly.) Pin facing to neck edge. When you come to collar, turn back shoulder seam allowance of facing and baste to itself, not to bodice. Make double bias cut 2 in. wide, or wider, and place over collar at back neck stitches. Have about 1/4 in. of double bias extend beyond stitches in bodice area and 1/4 in. beyond shoulder seam at top of facing. Baste all in position.

All parts of neck are now firmly basted in place and you can proceed without worrying about anything shifting. Turn the whole neck unit over so you can see all your previous stitches. **6.** The inside of the garment is upward. Stitch slowly from folded edge to folded edge on regular seam allowance. Make sure you don't accidentally catch in some part underneath. It's a help to put a piece of newsprint under the end where you start stitching to aid in putting the needle very near the fold, (X). Tear away paper.

7. Tie threads where you started and stopped. Select a very fine needle and thread it with one thread-end. Send it head first under first one stitch and then another. Clip thread. Do the same with its mate. Repeat process for other thread-ends. **8.** Stitch entire neck again, close row of stitches, ch. 6. Dispose of thread-ends as before. Trim very close to stitches and coat with sealant. Remove bastings at neck and front fold. Turn.

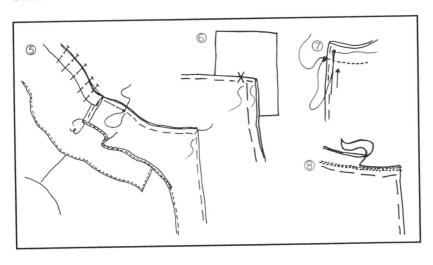

9. Working with inside of neck toward you, pin and then baste bodice/facing fold to hold in its final position. Baste neck to hold seam up in its permanent position. As you reach collar area, manipulate with your fingers to push collar upward to its fullest exposure. Baste just under seam. **10.** Place on table, inside of garment upward. Pin facing in position to bodice but don't baste. You will now probably need to remove bastings from little shoulder facing seam and change its slope slightly to agree with slope of bodice shoulder seam and be the same width. Trim as required and coat with sealant. **11.** Sew to shoulder seam by hand using small stitches. Don't go through to front of garment. Baste facing in place. Stitch near fold of bias overlapping facings slightly at shoulders. Fasten thread-ends.

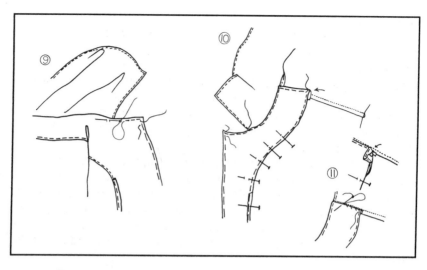

Turn bodice right side up. **12.** Cut a piece of newsprint large enough to go under entire front facing fold and front facing that needs to be sewn to bodice. Pin securely in place making sure front fold is perfectly straight. The newsprint keeps the bodice from rippling where stitches are on the bias. If you have a computerized machine, use Solvy. You can put the facing down by hand, in which case you don't need newsprint; take close-together stitches. Or, you may leave facings free from clips downward. Buttons and buttonholes will hold them in place.

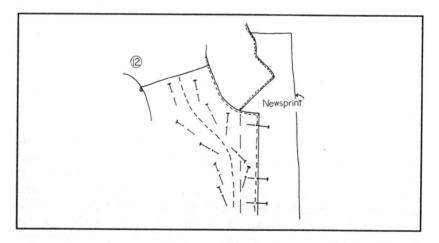

#11 BODICE WITH SIMPLE REVERS (fig. 7-10)

"Revers" is a corruption of the French word meaning reverse. You turn the front neck portion of this bodice back so you can see the reverse side of it. This easy answer to a collar is also the lapel part of the tailored collar. If you intend to add ornamentation, such as a ruffle as shown in this explanation, follow these general procedures. It requires a seam on the fold-line and the SHEER LAPEL, described earlier, has none.

Mount the bodice front and back sheers on lining fabric. (See ch. 9 for interesting ways to use chiffon in a situation such as this.) Cut two sets of front facings from sheer (or one layer of lining, whatever you've decided after reading ideas in ch. 9). **1.** Open out one set on table, right sides up. Put other set on top, right sides together. (Only one set will be described, but always work in pairs, mirror image, so you don't make two for one side and none for the other.) Pin all around and then baste across shoulder and down curving side leaving free at neck, down front and across bottom. **2.** Sew on machine on required seamline using very fine stitches, and clip off corner near stitches. Clip curved edge a place or two; you may grade seam. Turn right side out, baste near stitched edges and press. Join raw edges. Set aside.

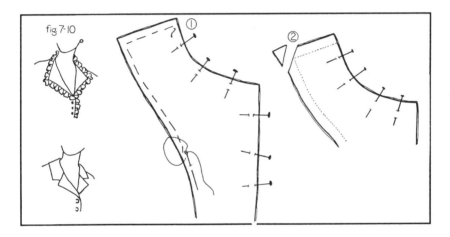

fig 7-10

3. If you want something like a ruffle, now is the time to pin it at the edge of the right side of bodice and baste in place. Double bias cut about 5 in. wide and folded (but not pressed!) down its length makes an attractive width ruffle for a 5/8 in. seam. At the point of revers, pin out of the way of future stitching. **4.** Baste the prepared facings on top of any trimming. If you have used a combination of sheer and lining for the facing, for this step the lining goes upward and the sheer touches the bodice. At back neck baste double bias overlapping facing at shoulders.

5. Stitch around neck and down fronts. Snip off corner and clip curve of neck as required to facilitate turning. **6.** Turn to inside and baste near edges to hold in position. Stitch bias from shoulder seam to shoulder seam. By hand sew facing to shoulder seam, not going through to the bodice. Remove basting from back of neck.

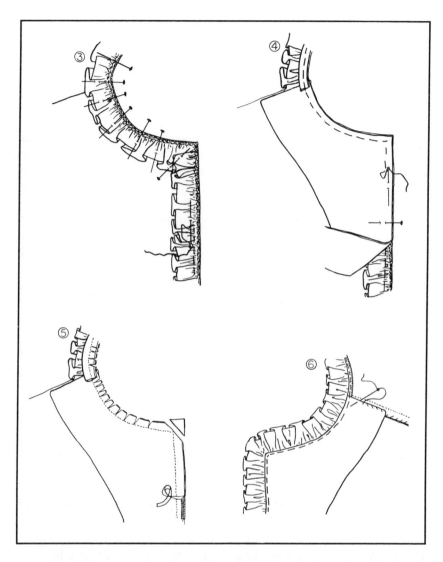

If you're sewing with a stiff sheer, press seams and leave in bastings until after you've made buttonholes. If you're sewing with a soft sheer, don't remove bastings from around revers even after you make buttonholes. Do not press. The idea is to let the bastings do the pressing for you. When the garment is totally finished you will examine it to judge what it needs in the way of pressing -- none, we hope.

#12 SPECIAL NECKLINE TREATMENTS, SHEER GARMENT (fig. 7-11)

Let these general suggestions guide you in as you are confronted with the unusual.

Follow the steps in the pattern directions about joining any special type "collar". Decide whether or not to interface (using the desired amount of stiffness or softness) following the appropriate ideas in the #8

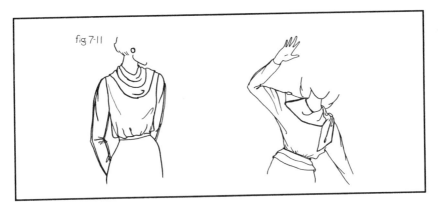

fig 7-11

FLAT COLLAR and #14 BUTTONHOLE paragraphs. Finish the raw edges of each interior seam. The fine zigzag rolled edge is a good choice.

CAMISOLE

Although you can get by with it in casual clothes, it's otherwise unsuitable to have buttons on the front bodice of a garment and behind this have buttons on a camisole, too. If you don't want to wear a separate camisole which you simply tuck into your skirt, there is an answer. Suppose your garment opens in the front, will have elastic at the waist and the bodice has no extra blousing at the center front. Split the pattern on the center front line and add seam allowance to match that of the sheer garment. After you've finished the top and side seams of the camisole, lay its center fronts against those of the bodice; include the camisole in the construction of the bodice.

#13 CAMISOLE OPENS IN BACK (fig. 7-12)

If bodice opens in back, whether zipper or buttons, camisole must also open in the back. Sometimes camisole, after being split down center, can be sewn in with bodice. But if it needs to have a separate placket in back, these paragraphs tell you what to do.

Cut camisole out of lining fabric following altered pattern. Overcast side edges of front and backs, back facings and center backs. Position straps to front and construct camisole front. If there's a separate facing across top of back camisole, sew it in place and press seam open. Side seams are not yet joined, but the top of front is complete.

1. Pin the correct length of elastic 1/4 in. to 3/8 in. wide (that won't be harmed by machine-stitches) at side, so it will be caught in side-seam stitches.   Machine-stitch end of elastic to hold.   **2.** Fold self-facing near center back on new fold line. Pin other end of elastic so it lacks 1/2 in. of reaching fold. Machine-stitch end of elastic. **3.** Fold back facing down and pin so elastic is held out of harm's way while you sew facing to camisole with a small running stitch. **4.** Sew side seams and turn toward front. **5.** Sew hook and eye at top (the 1/2 in. where elastic doesn't reach). Put more hooks and eyes or Velcro dots down to within 2 in. from waist. Sew straps in position in back.

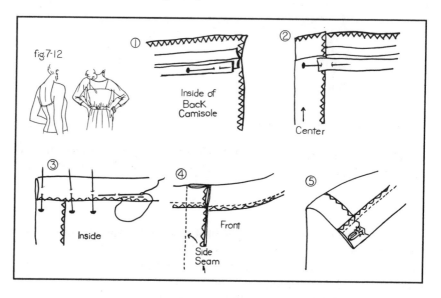

Set aside and await further developments which follow after you've installed zipper or buttons in back of bodice. See ch. 8.

DETAILS

#14 BUTTONHOLES AND BUTTONS (fig. 7-13)

If you know the placement, it's easier to make buttonholes before you set in the sleeves, if any. However, if you're not sure how to proceed with any special handling with the base of the placket, you must put off buttonhole- making until later. A shirt presents no problems because it terminates in a hem.

Buttonholes are no harder to make in sheers than on any other cloth if you use proper materials as dependable assistants. The following suggestions are for two layers of chiffon that have no interfacing in the construction. You face such a situation when the sheer bodice with folded-back self-facing is coupled with the sheer collar. From the sheerest to the least transparent, you need only adapt to your special situation, and the solution may be exactly the same. For the two layers of only chiffon, have buttonholes no longer than 5/8 in. long. Although the buttonhole itself is fairly strong, there is no extra support above or below, allowing a longer buttonhole to fall open.

As for the buttons, you have another concern besides the size and that's the weight. Don't pull down the bodice with heavy buttons no matter how beautiful. For example, some with rhinestones are gorgeous but weigh a ton. None of these sheers look good when heavy buttons drag down the area. For the more sporty look you can use a smooth 2 or 4-hole shirt button, the lightweight ball or half-ball button or something similar. For the dressier sheer you may use the half-ball in the appropriate color as well as the small stud-like rhinestone or very small half-ball in gold. The sheer garment is beautiful. Don't gild the lily.

Turn finished bodice with facing upward. Down length of buttonhole area pin a strip of organza (the same color or lighter), wider than that required for buttonhole. Because of fragility of cloth, run buttonholes across as shown so button will pull against the buttonhole's greatest strength. Turn garment over. On right side down the same area, place a strip of transparent stabilizer such as Solvy. Pin and then baste all layers together. Mark buttonholes on Solvy with disappearing ink and then make machine buttonholes. With your fine scissors, trim organza close to machine-stitches. Do the same for the Solvy in front.

Even for heavier sheers when you use an interfacing this exact method will no doubt be all you need; but should you want a firmer base, use two layers of organza.

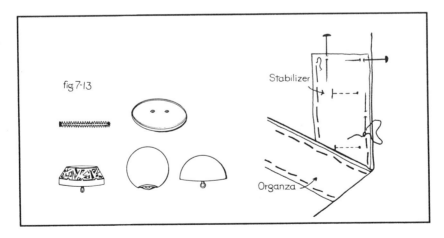

fig 7-13

Stabilizer

Organza

Master the art of making machine buttonholes in cotton cloth so you feel completely at ease with your buttonhole maker. Know where to lower the needle at the start for exact placement -- buttonholes are always difficult to pick out, but you're not going to get away with it in a sheer.

Don't make buttonholes by hand unless you're a past master. If poorly done your garment screams, "Homemade!"

#15 PATCH POCKET (fig. 7-14)

If you've ever struggled making, placing and attaching a patch pocket to a front bodice and then uttered the disappointing truth, "I can hardly see it!" you know why you seldom bother putting a patch pocket on a patterned cloth. Instead, it should be the one decorative detail to give a garment distinction. The patch pocket is the only type suitable for sheers. What follows is the best method for making a pocket for the sheerest cloth. The more opaque your fabric, the more likely it is you can use standard patch pocket construction.

Save an area for your pocket when you cut out. When ready to sew pocket to garment, cut it out roughly more than 1 in. bigger than you want it. Then pull threads to make it the correct finished size + about an inch on sides and bottom, and allowing for double (deep) hem at top. Cut absolutely on grain. **1.** Make the double hem in the top.

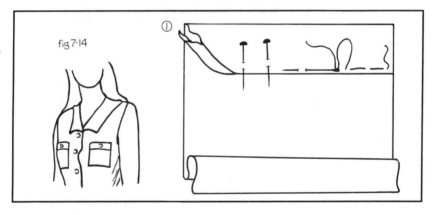

fig 7-14

2. Starting at the upper right-hand corner and using the presser foot or an attachment as a guide, stitch the very fine zigzag around the three sides of the pocket. Trim very close to stitches, but don't clip one. **3.** Now is the time to make a buttonhole in the center of the double hem if you want one.

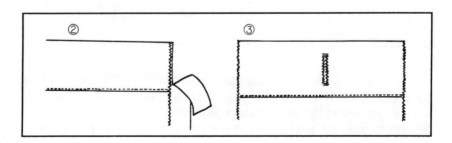

4. Hand-baste edge toward back 1/8 in. to 3/16 in. **5.** Hand-baste to bodice front and sew in place by hand more or less invisibly. The ideal width of the turn-under is the width of the garment's shoulder seams.

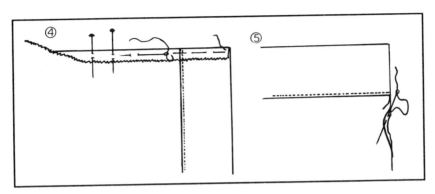

For the sporty dress or shirt, you can cut a rectangle allowing for the double hem at the top and about 3/8 in. around the sides and bottom. You may snip off a little at the corners. Turn the edges in twice 3/16 in. and stitch twice to the bodice -- once on the very edge and once inward about 3/16 in.

To put something in the sheer pocket would spoil it. It's all for show.

#16 BIG DART (fig. 7-15)

Sew dart, continuous thread method.   **1.** Trim to about 1/2 in. **2.** Fold one side inward until raw edge almost touches stitches. Fold in other edge, also. **3.** Sew the two sides together by hand or machine. Try

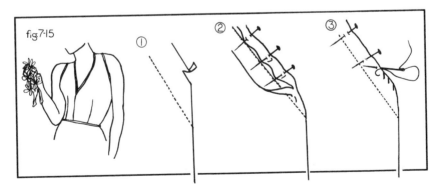

fig 7-15

to have the resulting "seam" about the same width as the side seams or shoulder seams.

If the area that has the big dart is mounted, make the dart in the usual fashion and overcast the raw edges.

SLEEVES

If you fitted your garment correctly in the muslin, you know the armhole is perfectly placed and the sleeve the correct length for the chosen finish.

#17 CONTINUOUS STRIP PLACKET (fig. 7-16)

Not all sleeves need a placket, but we show this one because it works in conjunction with the cuff presented later.

This simple placket is perfect for sheers. If you've had poor luck with it in the past, put your fears to rest; it's one of the easiest methods if you know what to do. In this example the placket is sewn in the left sleeve before the underarm is sewn or the sleeve set in. It's much easier to handle and you won't muss the body of the garment.

1. Make a dot 2 in. or less from the bottom of the sleeve in the proper place, usually on the back quarter. The placket is short because it only needs to open wide enough to allow your hand to pass through. Cut to within 1/8 in. of dot. Cut a strip of sheer 1-in. wide or less.

The first method is from the outside of sleeve. **2.** Hold right side of sleeve toward you. Without basting, sew strip in place by hand taking minute stitches a scant 1/4 in from edge. Take a little backstitch every few

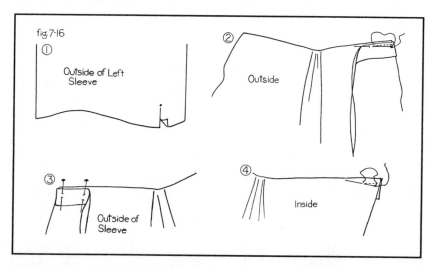

fig 7-16

① Outside of Left Sleeve

② Outside

③ Outside of Sleeve

④ Inside

stitches. When you reach dot, narrow seam to about 1/8 in. You will no doubt make a small pleat in the sleeve. This is hard to avoid, but don't give it a thought. If your stitches are tiny the pleat will be tiny, too.

3. For the second method again start strip on outside but at the other end. Put a pin in to hold and turn to inside of sleeve. **4.** Sew on the strip the same way. You may find it easier to cope with the area near the dot.

5. With inside of sleeve toward you, baste under the other edge of strip about 1/4 in. and sew to the seam allowance by hand. Make your stitches very small and about 1/16 in. apart. When you reach the dot again, you will probably think you can never get the strip on properly, that you will cause some puckering. Just keep going and if your stitches are very small, all will be well. Remove bastings.

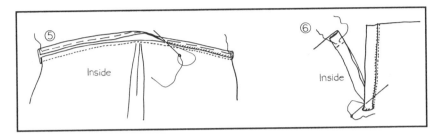

The finish is just as important as the rest and many a seamstress has made a mistake after doing everything else perfectly. **6.** Here's what you do: EXTEND THE BUTTON END AND FOLD BACK THE BUTTONHOLE END. Fold and baste in those positions at the wrist in preparation for the cuff. Tack placket to itself in that position on the inside near the dot. And which, you ask, is the button end? It is the one nearer the underarm seam. Please take special notice of this because IF you do this right, and IF you label the sheer pieces correctly after the cut-cut, and IF you lay the right side of the cuff against the right side of the sleeve matching notches when you sew on the cuff, THEN you cannot have the cuffs lap the wrong direction. This has plagued every seamstress since cuffs came into being.

Do not press. Now you sew underarm seam.

Employ the foregoing system using French piping when you want to open the neck where the garment has no seam.

#18 CUFF (fig. 7-17)

The sleeve placket is complete and underarm seam sewn. Handle the cuff for the sporty version in the same fashion as you did #9, SHIRT COLLAR WITH COLLARBAND AND FRONT BAND. See ch. 9 for another finish at the wrist. The cuff presented now is a standard version without topstitching. You may use lining for interfacing or a soft woven type; but interfacing and thread must match the sheer.

Open out the two cuff linings on table wrong sides up. (Only the one for the left sleeve will be illustrated hereafter, but do both the same way, mirror image.) If you haven't marked the fold line, do so now. **1.** Trim two corners from interfacing as shown and place against fold line.

If your sheer has a pattern or if it is as opaque as Georgette, you stitch the four sides like this: stitch 1/8 in. away from fold; on the three other

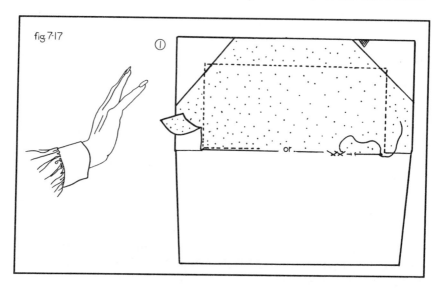

fig 7-17

①

sides, stitch 3/4 in. from edge. Trim close to stitching. But, if it is glass-clear, cross- stitch fold-edge going through only the interfacing with a small stitch; the other small stitch is IN the fold. Only baste sleeve/cuff edge; it will be caught in with that seam. Stitch the cuff ends 3/4 in. from edge as above. Trim near ends.

Turn this unit over so interfacing is down and mount sheer to it. Probably a little sheer extends here and there beyond lining; trim to size of lining.

2. Fold cuff on fold line, right sides together; the interfacing is exposed. Pin ends together. Notice that the underside of cuff seems too small; later it will be all right. Stitch ends of cuff. Trim the two corners near the fold. Turn cuff right side out. Put gathering threads in end of sleeve using the big machine-stitch, or by hand, starting and stopping at placket. Place one row 3/8 in. from edge and other row 3/4 in. from edge. 3. With right sides together pin sleeve to cuff matching notches. Draw up gathering threads to cuff size and figure 8 around end pins. Spread out the gathers evenly. Pin, baste carefully and stitch. 4. Baste the layers of seam allowance through interfacing and lining to front of cuff. Continue basting seam allowance in extension. Do not remove gathering threads in the seam allowance.

5. With under-cuff upward, fold cuff near fold line (you can feel where interfacing reaches) and smooth cuff toward unsewn edge. Turn under that edge the amount required to stop short of sleeve/cuff stitchline and pin to seam allowance. It appears that the seam of cuff/sleeve is much

too large, that gaps and puckers are present. It will be correct when finished. Gently ease to fit putting a smidgen more ease at each end near

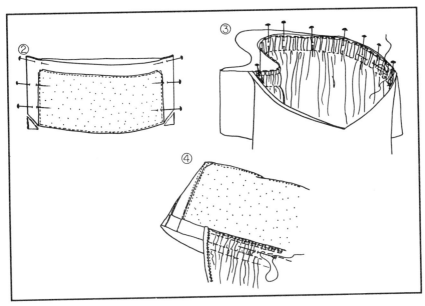

placket than elsewhere. Sew by hand. Do NOT ease in upper cuff to fit; have hand stitches about 3/16 or 1/4 in. apart and let it loop between stitches. Fasten thread occasional. This allows cuff to curve around wrist.
6. With right side of cuff toward you, baste ends of cuff rolling the under-side so it doesn't show.

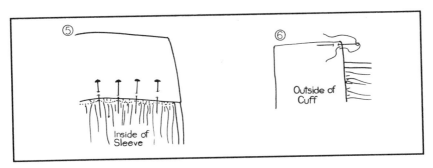

Do not press. Do not remove bastings until after you make buttonholes or sew on snaps.

This cuff has it all. It shows no stitching on the right side and no heavy color of seams at edges. It is gently yet completely supported by what means no one knows. And it curves nicely around the wrist with no extra cloth from underneath fighting to expose itself.

We now resume the exciting mystery of the mounted yoke. As you recall from the last episode, bodices were joined to their linings and these in turn were sewn to mounted yokes. Shoulder seams were made and the completed facings were waiting. All was in readiness. Only the sleeves delayed the action. We rejoin the story for the exciting conclusion of the MYSTERY OF NO VISIBLE SUPPORT FOR THE

#19 MOUNTED YOKES, PART II (fig. 7-18)

Put gathering threads in cap of sleeve. **1.** With right sides together, pin sleeve to bodice. Holding yoke out of the way, join sleeve to bodice through underarm using very fine stitches. Start stitching at arrow and pass through spot where you terminated yoke/bodice stitching. Stitch again employing the two rows of stitches. **2.** With right sides together, pin sleeve to yoke drawing up gathering threads to fit. You almost have to turn the little armscye seam toward sleeve in this situation. Stitch in place securing stitches at dots. Don't remove gathering threads from seam allowance. **3.** Baste seam allowance to wrong side of yoke. Clip more if required.

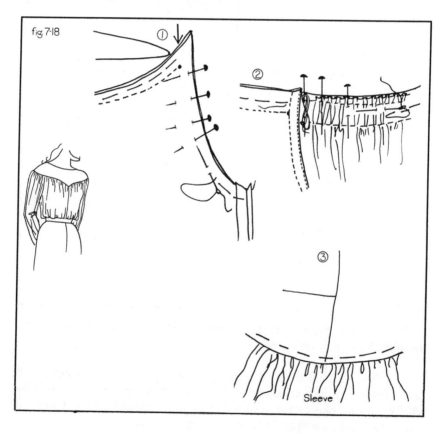

fig 7-18

① ② ③

Sleeve

Remove paper stay and staystitch neck using very fine stitches 1/32 in. less than the 5/8 in. seam allowance. Fold bodice back into finished position for buttons or zipper, whatever you've planned. (When finished, back yoke edge will equal turn-back of back bodice.

4. Pin prepared yoke lining in position, right sides together, joining the backs, around neck and down other back to yoke/bodice seam. Baste. Turn over and machine-stitch so you can see the staystitching on Georgette neck which will be just barely to your right. Later, it will be out of sight. 5. Trim neck and clip as required to lie flat. Trim off corners at back neck. Turn right side out. 6. Baste all around the just-completed seam, holding right side toward you and roll facing out of sight. On wrong side smooth yoke facing toward yoke/bodice seam and pin occasionally including such places as center front and notches. By hand sew just inside seam allowance with small stitches.

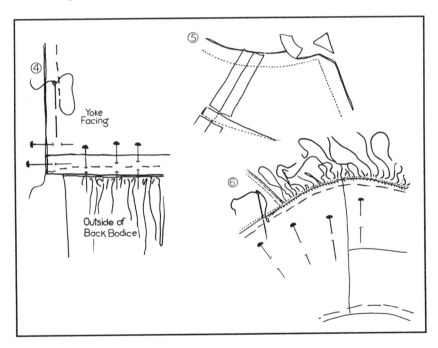

This system works well for yokes for any fabric when you want facings to stay where the belong -- out of sight. It solves THE MYSTERY OF NO VISIBLE SUPPORT FOR THE MOUNTED YOKE.

Have you waited all this time wondering how to finish the yoke/sleeve seam when you have a sheer yoke? Well, it was mentioned earlier, but we'll repeat it. You always bind the yoke/bodice seam with bias when there are gathers. Then set in the sleeves. Next, bind the entire armscye with bias if the sheer is as clear as glass. If the cloth is more opaque and there are no gathers in the top of sleeve, use the turned and stitched seam finish for the sleeve cap and the two rows of stitches finish under the arm from notches to notches.

In most cases you now assemble the layers of the bodice, matching side seams and other cardinal places. You are ready for the skirts.

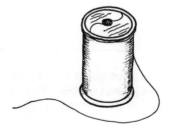

8

SEWING FROM THE WAIST DOWN

In this chapter we tackle sewing from the waist down, which includes such things as making and handling the skirt layers, joining them to the bodice if there's a waist seam, openings down the back, and hems. Although these things are often bulky and take time, you have already done much of the exacting work. The garment is well underway.

If you're making a shift, you had to sew the side seams before you handled the armholes. But if there is a waist seam, it is time to sew the panels of the skirt. Use the seams that are most appropriate to your fabric as suggested in ch. 6. Sew underskirt seams at this time, too.

Sounds easy, but what do you do if the sewing of the skirt seams is baffling? Read the following paragraphs to find answers to special situations.

#1 THE DEEP HEM

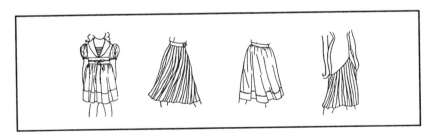

In ch. 6 you saw the mechanics of sewing the deep hem. However, unlike other hems, you put this one in before you join the skirt to the bodice. This holds true for skirts made from border print fabric, skirts made with horizontal tucks near the hem and similar decoration. (This is not the same as something you sew on top of the cloth after the skirt is finished, such as ribbon.) But, before you can sew this hem, you have to sew the side seams and the center back (or wherever it opens) past the hem and almost to where you judge the placket to start.

A similar situation exists when you send fabric off to be pleated, except you can't finish the job. You join enough panels to go around your hips comfortably when the pleats are closed; hem. Then, when you receive the pleated product, you do the final joining, which is usually in the center back. Before you consider the details of joining the pleats correctly, see how you get the bottom of the skirt equidistant from the floor.

Little girls who measure about the same at the waist and hips have no problem. Mother simply allows for the correct depth hem and makes the skirt accordingly. The same holds true for a woman with very modest curves. But an adult with a noticeable swell at the hips or abdomen handles the skirt differently. Follow these steps after you have already put in the deep hem. Put on the shoes you will wear with the skirt.

#2 GATHERED STRAIGHT SKIRT (fig. 8-1)

Draw on the skirt and have your friend tie a string around your waist, exactly placed. This is the waist stitchline. It helps to slip a wide strip of soft paper, such as tissue paper, inside next to your skin. First, place the center back opening. Then, your friend arranges the gathers attractively for your figure. The 3-in. extra you added when you cut out will extend unevenly above the string. Your friend will adjust the hem by keeping her eye on how it measures at the bottom. If it is too long at one spot, she pulls the skirt up above the string a bit until it is correct at the hem. If it is too short, she tugs the skirt down a bit more as necessary.

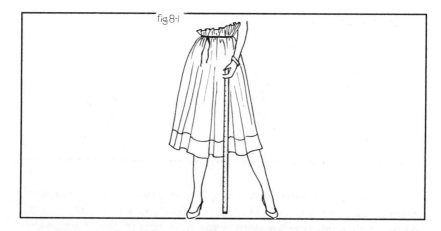
fig. 8-1

When the entire hem hangs perfectly according to the yardstick, she re-checks the gathers at the string. When all is well, she slips her fingers under the paper and pins in the gathers at the string-line to the paper, positioning correctly and then noting on the paper the centers and sides. Remove skirt and baste gathers in place going through paper, too. Add seam allowance and trim away excess. Tear away paper before you proceed.

If this skirt is chiffon, you need a chiffon underskirt. Prepare it, too, and set both aside until you are ready to assemble the skirt layers.

#3 PLEATED SKIRT (fig. 8-2)

Sew Back Seam The example has 1/2 in. pleats that go to the right. The size of the pleat determines the amount of overlap you must have. However, the location of the seam that joins the pleated fabric is the important thing. It is better if this joining seam is very slightly to the right of center back. This means the overlap is to the right of that. If you keep this fact in the back of your mind as you work that's all you need to do now. Later, you can shift the pleated skirt a bit to position it precisely when you actually sew it to the bodice or band. Your body shape won't vary noticeably in one inch.

1. Measure up from bottom of hem to what you judge to be the fullest part of hip and baste pleats closed there. Pleating should appear to be uninterrupted at overlap. The overlap requires at least 1 1/4 in. to fold back to act as a facing. The underlap also needs 1 1/4 in. but for it you *extend* the extra cloth. Press pleats out of both of these extensions. Trim away extra cloth when you see just how much you need for placket. The ideal place to join the pleats is in an inward fold so when the skirt opens the join will look unnoticeable. You start this process at the hip level. Do not incorporate any extra pleats; only the placket requires that.

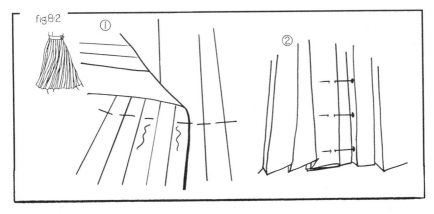

2. Follow this joining to hem pinning as you go. This is important because you want to work on the same pleats at both places.

3. Lift up upper layer. Arrow points to start of stitching. To repeat, the perfect place to make this join is where the cloth would have an inward fold were there no seam; the skirt looks attractive when pleats swing open. Carry machine stitching to start of placket. The very flat two rows of stitches is a good finish for this seam. Trim from bottom to within 1 in. of placket. Coat seam with sealant after the trimming.

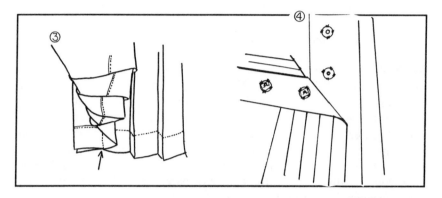

Even the Hem Tie the string around the waist, arranging the pleats so they overlap a little where the lower body swells the most; you want the final effect to be one of pleats going from the waist straight down to the floor. If pleats have to fall open to go over a larger area, they won't look right. If the fabric is soft like chiffon, use a combination of overlapping and easing. Soft fabric can manage to absorb as much as 13 in. and still not look gathered. Proceed as for GATHERED SKIRT to even hem. Carefully remove the skirt. If you machine baste the pleats to tissue paper, go the direction of the pleating. Measure for the seam allowance at waist and it's ready to join the lining. The pleated skirt does not need another layer of sheer.

Sew snaps   4. Snaps are appropriate to a sheer because they are lightweight. Sew them to overlap facing going through only one layer of sheer. Position snap so it is under the fold of the next pleat, in this case back more than 1/2 in. Sew on several about 1 1/2 in. apart stopping short of the waist seam about 1 1/2 in. Sew on their mates. They need to appear neat from the outside of pleated skirt, which is different from your usual concern.

#4 UNDERSKIRT FOR BELTED SHIFT (fig. 8-3)
You have already sewn the side seams and center back seams of lining and sheer as explained in 7-2. You marked the waist in 3-6, step 3. (If there are no gathers necessitating the last step, mark waist now.) Press side seams to hems. Press center back seams as follows from low hip level

to hem: the lining open, the sheer seam one direction and the underskirt the opposite direction. Press side seams. Don't fasten off threads at base of placket opening.

Place garment on table. Fold the chiffon dress skirt up toward the shoulders to expose the marked waistline of lining. From the hem slide the prepared underskirt up toward the waist and pull its lower edge up toward the shoulders, also. **1.** Underskirt is now wrong side out. Put raw edge of waist 1/2 in. below waistline mark. Match center front and the stitchlines of side seams. Match center back lines and raw edges.

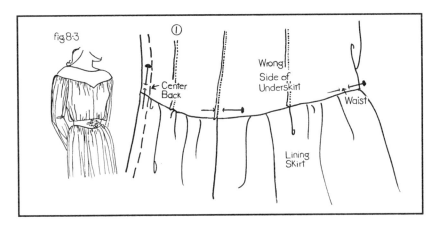

2. Lining and underskirt will not be the same size so take little tucks in one to be the same size as the other. Place tucks from side front to side back on each half of the garment, or as you have found to be flattering to your body. With large zigzag stitches, go over raw edge of underskirt. Stitch again using regular length stitches on the waistline mark. Pull underskirt down and smooth at waist seam. Stitch again either zigzag stitch or regular stitch. Seam will be hidden by belt.

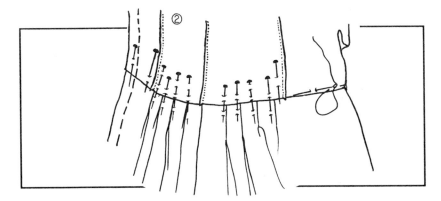

If you think your underskirt is heavy and will weigh down the lining, raise the application 1/2 in. You don't want the stitches that join the underskirt to lining to show below the belt -- nor above the belt, either.

#5 DRESS WITH LOW WAISTLINE (fig. 8-4)

In this example the bodice lining will not hang free but will be connected to the bodice and flounce at the low waistline. The bodice may or may not be partially connected in the upper regions; it makes no difference in the procedure described here. Of course, both flounce and bodice must measure the same at the seam and bodice lining must be the correct length.

Baste sheer(s) and bodice lining together at low waistline, matching notches, seams and centers. **1.** Make satin-stitch dot exactly where seams cross at peak of center front skirt (see 7-3, 1 and 2). Set aside. **2.** With cut-out pleated fabric still attached to newsprint flounce pattern, pin more closely and machine-baste above and below proposed seamline at top. Stitch the same direction as the pleats. (If required, place Solvy over pleats to protect them). Tear paper away. (The hem was sewn in before you had fabric pleated.)

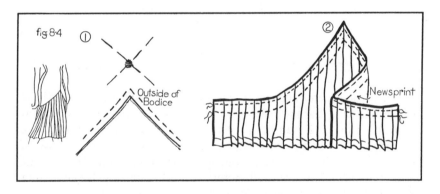

3. Completely construct flounce lining. Because of the bias nature of the front flounce area, you must stabilize it to keep low bodice and flounce from stretching at the seam. Pin front lining *pattern* on the right side of lining. On wrong side pin and then stitch matching seam tape, or other stabilizing tape, over seamline so it will barely be caught in the stitching; it extends into seam allowance no more than 1/8 in. Tear paper pattern away after application. If your machine is computerized, handle flounce lining very carefully and apply tape; see 7-6. **4.** Place pleated sheer over flounce lining and start pinning in place at top, edges even. Notice, both fabrics are right side upward. As you near the center back, judge the best possible place to join pleats. See 8-3 for joining method. If you have a little extra pleated fabric to ease in, spread it over as much of back area as possible. View from outside to check final appearance. Baste the layers of this flounce affair by hand. Machine-stitch.

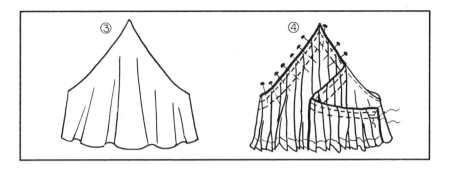

    5. Clip bodice up to satin-stitch dot. You may pin and stitch the little portion there just as in 7-3, 7 and 8. Or, as you see here, start pinning and stitching at one center front; stitch that half and then stitch the other half of the flounce seam. Clip only as required, and test first.
6. Overcast resulting raw edges and baste seam allowances up against bodice. Press.

    If you choose a free-hanging bodice lining, bind bodice/flounce seam.

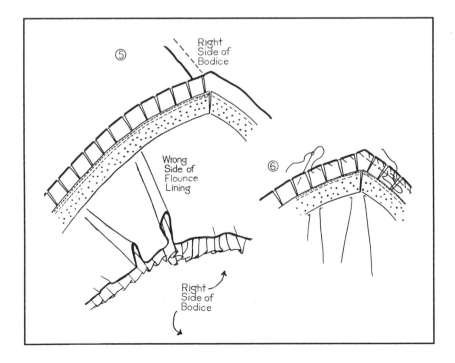

This example is one of the most difficult possible. Yours will probably be easier. If the waistline is only slightly dropped, handle as any other skirt you join to the bodice.

#6 DRESS WITH PARTIAL WAISTLINE (fig. 8-5)

The bodice of this dress is often mounted. First you sewed the darts in the bodice and "skirt" lining as suggested in 3-14. However, you have an interesting problem because, although you want the skirts hang free, you have no waist seam at sides and back to help you. In our example it is possible to make a French seam (or use another seam finish) on the center front seam of sheer skirt. Then, separately, sew the center front lining seam. Gather the sheer to match the darted lining and then sew the partial waistline seam joining bodice and skirt. The skirt now hangs free at center front.

1. In the mounting process of the bodice, stop the stitching of all other seams at a point equal to about 2 in. below the partial seam, point X. Backstitch or otherwise fasten threads well. Handle the center back seam as described in #7. **2.** With dress still wrong side out, pin the lining out of the way and insert the machine needle in the sheer at point X. Stitch seam to hem. Stitch again making the two rows of stitches finish. Secure the threads well at point X and weave them in the stitches if required to hide ends. Clip through seam allowance to point X and trim seam. Repeat for the remainder of sheer skirt seams. (You have already handled the center back seam.) **3.** With the dress still wrong side out, pin the sheer out of the way and stitch the lining seam with right sides together from X down to the hem. Repeat for remaining lining seams.

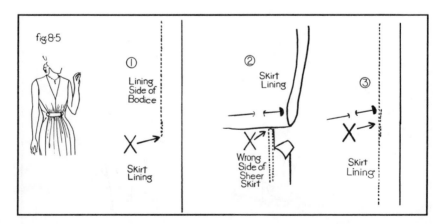

fig 8-5

① Lining Side of Bodice

Skirt Lining

② Skirt Lining

Wrong Side of Sheer Skirt

③ Skirt Lining

With the inside of the lining upward, slip the lining skirt over the ironing board. (The sheer skirt hangs off the board.) Press each seam open from very near point X to hem. Make sure sheer is out of the way.

Next, place sheer only on the ironing board, with the lining hanging off, and press those seams the way they want to lie. Finally, turn the garment right side out and slip both layers of skirt over board right side up. Feel underneath to make sure the lining seam is open and check to see that the sheer seam lies as pressed. Then press the right side at point X. Repeat for each seam. You do not have an underskirt with this type garment.

PUTTING IT ALL TOGETHER

You've make skirts, linings and in most cases you've assembled the layers for the bodice. Where do you go from here?

Unless there is a special situation such as those mentioned later under COMBINATIONS OF CLOSURES, it's time to stack the skirt layers and prepare to join them at the waist. If there is an underskirt (or more than one) put it over the lining. On top slip the sheer garment. All right sides are upward. Match side seams, centers and notches. Baste all together. With right sides together join to assembled bodice layers matching, again, side seams, centers and notches. If the bodice is sheer, bind the resulting seam but stop short of the placket. You will finish that part of waist seam after placket is complete. If bodice has an attached lining at the waist, you may only overcast if you wish.

#7 PREPARATION FOR CENTER BACK PLACKET IN A SEAM
(fig. 8-6)

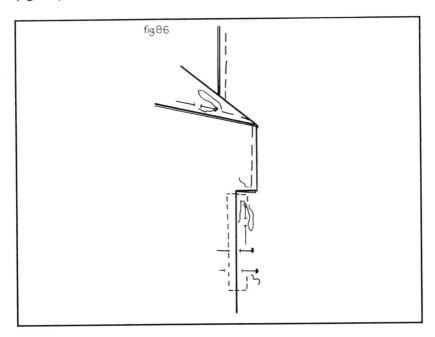

fig.8-6

Remeasure from neck, or waist, to the bottom of the opening on the sheer to see if it is the correct depth for your zipper (or other). A small amount of zipper tape will be included in neck finish. For no reason should you make the opening so small you must strain to pass it over your hips or shoulders. When depth is satisfactory, fasten threads in sheer strongly. Starting at the neck, pin all the layers of cloth together superimposing center back markings and matching waist seams (if any). Adjust other center back skirt seams to correspond in depth to the sheer. Either take out a few stitches or sew a few extra stitches by hand using thread-ends from the seam. Fasten all threads very well.

One at a time, clip the seam allowance of the sheer seam to stitchline. (For zipper you *may* not have to clip lining to center back seam.) If there's an underskirt, do the same to its seam. Press lining seam open. Press sheer seam one direction. If there's an underskirt, press its seam opposite to that of the upper sheer. Stack the layers so that the start of each opening is even and center back seamlines are exactly superimposed. Going through all layers of cloth, baste around the seam for about 3 in. to secure.

Although this exact method is not operational for the pleated sheer, it works for most situations, not just a zipper. Use it when the opening is in the seam and you have two or more layers of skirt which you want to hang free.

#8 ZIPPER IN CENTER BACK SEAM, MOUNTED CONSTRUCTION
Look at this one first because it is the most straightforward. If the bodice is partially or wholly mounted, install it exactly as you would for any opaque cloth after you prepare layers for a placket. If you saved an inch or two on either side of the center back neck to complete after you installed the zipper, you include a little bit of tape in this procedure. The stop is then about 1/8 in. below the finished neck. As a matter of fact, this is the neatest way to finish the top of the neck. The only change you may want to make is to do the top stitching on overlap by hand. Do the stitching on other side of zipper teeth by hand or machine.

#9 ZIPPER IN SHEER CLOTH (fig. 8-7)
This pertains particularly to chiffon. You have cut seam allowance 1 in. wide, as suggested in ch 5.

You have this situation when the procedure is partly concealed behind the many skirt layers, yet revealed in the bodice where you have a camisole with a separate closure. Try to avoid having the entire zipper installed in a completely sheer area if chiffon. For moderately loose garments, use the CONTINUOUS STRIP PLACKET, ch. 7, if there is no seam; or use the BOUND PLACKET IN A SEAM presented in this chapter. Many sheers that are more opaque or more sturdy, such as gauze, can handle the zipper without reinforcement.

The center installation in unmounted chiffon is poor because the cloth is all too easily ensnarled in the zipper teeth; there goes your dress. If your assistant in dressing is an impatient husband, think about this. Even with tape to give it body, it readily reveals the zipper teeth. From all the zipper installations you can choose, the lapped type, with modifications given here, is best for chiffon-only area.

Sew the seam together temporarily with machine bastings. **1.** Lay matching seam tape against temporary stitches and sew by machine on the very edge with very fine stitches. This important step gives the delicate cloth a bit of stability and protection. Fold chiffon over free side of tape and stitch or "glue" in place; trim chiffon if required. Press seam open. **2.** Open zipper, place face down with teeth against seam in seam allowance only, as shown, and machine baste. (On plastic zipper, teeth will not show from wrong side.)

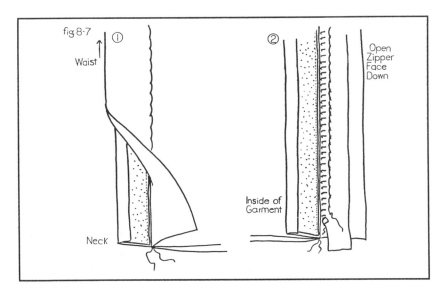

3. Close zipper, turn over and stitch next to new folded edge, still stitching only through seam allowance. **4.** Still on the wrong side, tug and smooth zipper to the left and baste in position. Fold edges of chiffon over tape and sew in place (to tape only) or "glue" with iron-on adhesive. Trim chiffon as needed. **5.** Instead of sewing second zipper stitching from the wrong side, turn over and stitch by hand using little backstitches. Of course, you can sew the other side by hand, too, instead of on machine. All raw edges are out of sight and no ragged edges will show. Remove bastings.

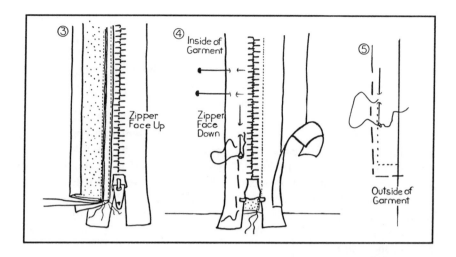

The trouble with all this is that even if you use the finest, narrowest, thinnest, most flexible zipper you can find, there is still a very wide heavy strip of color in delicate chiffon. Most zippers -- teeth and tapes -- measure about 1 in. or a little less. The only way to reduce that is trim some tape from each side and seal the raw edges. Narrow the chiffon accordingly as well as the reinforcing tape.

Another problem is the disposal of the zipper tape at the top. Place the zipper stops about 1/8 to 1/4 in. from proposed finished neck edge, and run the tape straight up and include some of it in the neck finish. Sew a hook and eye at the top.

#10 BOUND PLACKET IN A SEAM (fig. 8-8)

All yokes, seams, etc. must be joined. In this example the neck is already finished with a simple binding. Arrange the skirts as described in #7. Except for minor differences, upper and under plackets are made the same until you sew them together at the bottom. Both are the same width, but the upper part is bound with French piping and the lower with a straight-cut band. The center backs are superimposed when the placket is closed.

Upper Placket This center back placket is evenly divided on either side of the center back. Decide on the width of the finished placket. **1.** Put half of this to the left of center back and half to the right in the seam allowance at both the neck and base of placket. Mark with dots. This seam allowance remains on the right side even when placket is finished. Trim to pass through the right-hand dot if necessary, as illustrated. **2.** Baste French piping to the outside of garment so about 5/8 in. extends above neck and beyond opening at bottom. The stitchline will run from upper left dot down to lower left dot. Machine stitch, stopping even with the base of placket. As you near the bottom, hold other layers out of the way. Backstitch or otherwise secure well.

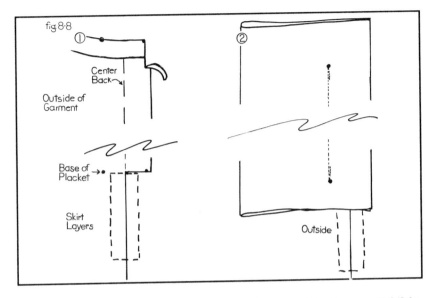

3. Trim extra French piping from the top and bottom until 3/8 in. remains; baste to itself to hold.

4. On wrong side, pin French piping for hand sewing. Draw top folds together with small stitches and continue to base of placket.

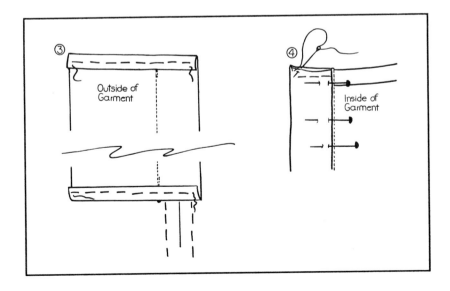

Under Placket The directions are almost the same -- except mirror image. Use a straight-cut strip of chiffon for the binding which you baste on the outside of the dress but stitch from the inside. **5.** Pin upper placket out of the way. This second seam allowance forms the foundation for the under placket and remains underneath the other part of placket when finished. Make the termination point 1/16 in. up from the base of placket. Handle hand-stitching as you did for the upper placket. **6.** On the right side of garment sew by hand across the bottom of the French piping catching in at least the chiffon garment. Don't attempt to sew through all layers and certainly not the under placket, which would be too bulky. Do this as "invisibly" as possible. **7.** Turn garment to the inside and tack the underbinding at the bottom. Remove center thread markers. Do not press if chiffon. Press other fabrics. Sew matching hook and eye at neck and at places of strain, with snaps in between; see ch. 10 for suggestions.

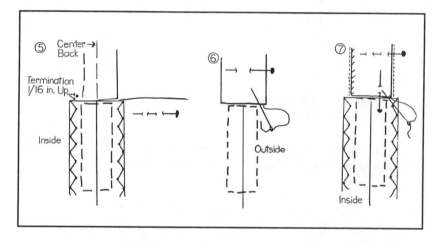

#11 SET-IN BAND WITH INVISIBLE ZIPPER (fig. 8-9)
    The Invisible zipper can be used in the seam under the arm if the bodice is mounted and has the standard set-in sleeve, and if the fit is moderately snug. Use the regular 5/8 in. seam allowance.
    The only difference in setting in the band is that you mount several layers of sheer to the set-in band before you proceed. You will, of course, face the band. Here are very brief directions. Leave the left side seam open appropriately. With right sides together, join the assembled layers of the bodice to the band, matching notches and seams and centers. On the inside of garment lay facing against bodice and join in the seam when you sew the bodice and band. Sew skirt layers to bottom of band, right sides together. By hand, sew band facing to band/skirt seam allowance. Use the instructions in #7 to prepare for the placket.

This closure is perfect for the sleeveless garment because the entire side opens up making it easy to put on. For the set-in sleeve, start the zipper about 1/2 in. down from armhole. (You must test in the trial

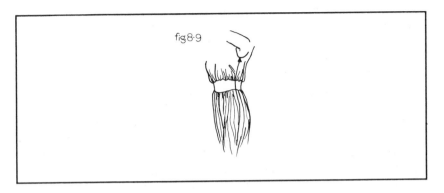

fig 8-9

garment to see if you can get it on over your shoulders.) No special installations instructions needed -- just follow the standard directions inclosed in the Invisible zipper folder.

COMBINATION OF BACK CLOSURES

What do you do when you have a combination of closures, sometimes one on top of another? In most cases it's hardly enough to tell the seamstress to "join at the waist". Here are rules to guide you.
1. Centers must match
2. No closure may interfere with another.
If you ask yourself these two questions when you're in doubt, and then experiment to see if you're really observing these rules, you can't go wrong. We'll look at two combination closures in depth.

#12 ATTACH CAMISOLE TO WAIST SEAM (fig. 8-10)
Although it looks quite lovely on the inside of a garment to do this attachment another way, it is hard to do and not necessary. How many people will see the inside of the waist seam -- the part next to your skin? Strength, serviceability and outside appearance are what count. So, we follow an easier path.

The camisole is cut the correct length and finished except for the bottom edge. With the exception of the hem, the sheer garment is complete and ready for the camisole. For clarification only, we have shortened the zipper in the skirt area. Although in reality you would have at least twice as much there, this is to help you see the relationship between the center back seam, the position of the zipper and the center of camisole layers.

1. Look at the zipper installation from the outside of the finished garment. The center back of skirt (or trousers) is the seam below the zipper stitches. **2.** From the inside of garment, looking only at zipper teeth and installation stitches and not at the base, it's hard to imagine that the center is not in the middle of the zipper teeth. However, you see that if you push a pin in at the base of zipper on the outside in the center back, it comes out at X in illustration 2.

To aid you in sewing camisole to waist seam, close zipper on sheer garment, turn the garment inside out and turn it end for end so the neck is closer to you on the table and the legs or skirts are smoothed out away from you toward the hems. **3.** Fasten camisole with its hooks, etc., and turn it, also, wrong side out. Slip it over shoulders of finished sheer garment and slide it down to waist. Match center front and side seams. Send a pin through the center back of camisole on waist seamline and through zipper tape center back. Slip fingers under zipper tape and seam allowance and clip camisole and seam allowance on the left at edge of zipper tape or overlap, whichever is farthest to the left. On the right clip at edge of zipper tape or overlap, whichever is farthest to the right.

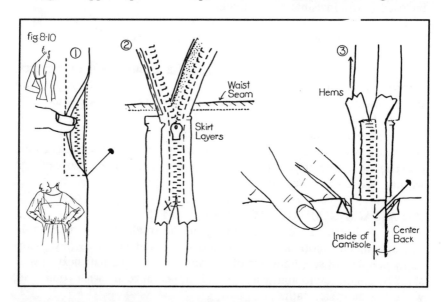

fig 8-10

① ② Waist Seam / Skirt Layers / X ③ Hems / Inside of Camisole / Center Back

4. From upper layer and then lower, trim about 1/4 in. from each little tab over zipper teeth and overcast each. Stitch each, one at a time, to itself. Pin camisole to waist/skirt seam all around and from the skirt side stitch 1/32 in. in seam allowance from other stitchline from clip to clip. **5.** Turn garment to right side and open zipper. Sew a dot of Velcro or a snap on very edge of camisole and its mate on zipper tape, as shown.

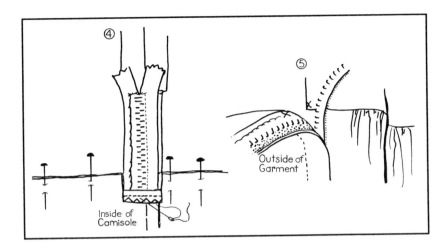

When you put on this garment, fasten back of camisole and then last little snap or Velcro dot before you zip up. If you like a real all-in-one garment, mount a bra inside camisole with straps, covered with the camisole fabric, acting as straps for both.

#13 PLEATED SKIRT WITH SNAPS, ZIPPER UNDERNEATH (fig. 8-11)

Let's look at the pleated skirt with snap closure coupled with the zipper in the lining that continues up into the bodice to the neck. This closure requires that the waistline bodice is lined just as if it were mounted. It can be a camisole that is sewn in with the bodice at the center back or something similar. Regardless, the bodice isn't sheer at the waist seam so the mechanics of the system are concealed. This procedure is not for the fainthearted.

This system requires that you finish neck after you sew waist seam and install zipper.

Preparation Join skirt lining at center back seam from base of placket upward with machine bastings but stop 1 1/2 in. from waist seam. Start installation of lapped zipper on the under side, steps 2 and 3 in fig. 8-7 but again stop about 1 1/2 in. from waist seam. Do not sew lapped side yet. Mark center back on both back skirt linings. At this point, skirt and lining aren't joined anywhere.

1. Mark on pleated skirt where skirt overlap reaches. By necessity, pleated skirt overlap is to the right of center; otherwise, the pleated skirt closure would interfere with the zipper. Center back on pleated skirt is approximately at the dotted line. Trim close to the snaps, turn under and stitch.

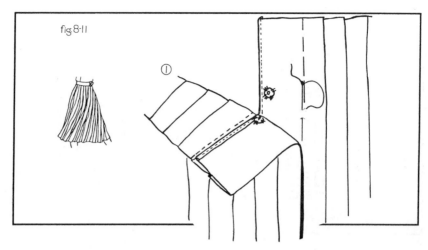

fig 8-11

2. Crease skirt lining on up to waist just as it will be when zipper is installed and lay its folded edge near zipper teeth. Place pleated skirt underlap on skirt lining near fold of lining in such a way that it will escape being caught in when you stitch lining to zipper tape. Open out seam allowance of lining at center back and pin pleated skirt to skirt lining on this underlap side only. Notice that you haven't pinned these layers to the zipper tape. Hold zipper and everything else out of the way while you stitch on machine, sewing pleated skirt underlap to skirt lining on seam line for about 3 in. 3. Making sure center back seam allowance of skirt lining is again opened out, place bodice on top of pleated skirt (and skirt lining) as shown, right sides together. Match center back of skirt lining and center back of bodice. Again, hold zipper and all else out of the way while you stitch waist seam. Stitch only 3 or 4 in. Press seam up against bodice. Refold lining on previous crease as seen in illustration 2 and stitch lining to zipper area. Complete the installation up to top of zipper on this side of zipper only. Don't catch in pleated skirt--it must hang free.

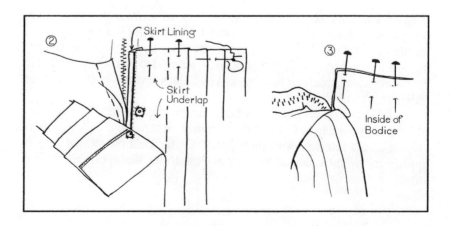

Skirt Lining

Skirt Underlap

Inside of Bodice

4. Fold pleated skirt overlap facing to the right side and stitch waist seam for about 4 in. **5.** Turn overlap facing to the inside (as it will be in the finished garment). Close zipper and fasten snaps.

> [Not shown: Lift pleated skirt, superimpose centers of skirt lining up toward waist seam. Fold seam allowance down on seamline so you can see to do the pin business. Smooth skirt back down in place.]

Put pin where you will stitch bodice overlap near zipper teeth as shown. Send a pin through all the layers and mark position on pleated skirt and lining. Mark on zipper tape, too, at waist seam.

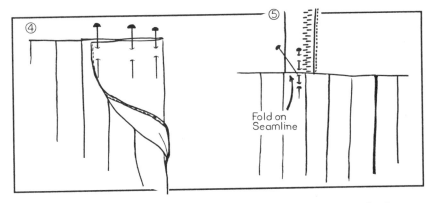

6. Turn overlap facing back to the front as before. Fold center back seam allowance of skirt lining the same direction as at base of placket and pin behind pleated skirt so skirt, lining and tape dots all match. **7.** Fold bodice back on its center back marks (lining against lining) and pin it on

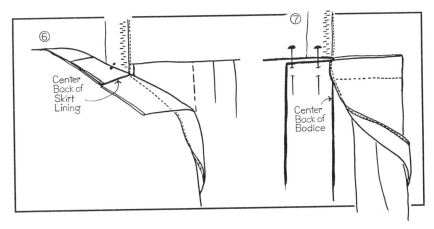

top of the pleated skirt with right sides together, in such a way that its center back is exactly superimposed on center back of the skirt lining. If necessary, bodice goes *under* overlap as shown.

(You notice that these centers are on folds.) Holding zipper and everything else out of the way, stitch on waist seamline for about 4 in. catching in skirts and bodice as shown. Fold overlap facing back to inside and all will be in place -- skirt layers down and bodice up in position.

8. Close zipper if open and fasten snaps. Baste and then pin bodice overlap in place; stitch to zipper tape on machine from waist to neck on right side as shown. **9.** Lift up pleated skirt and stitch lining to zipper tape from bottom of zipper to waist seam.

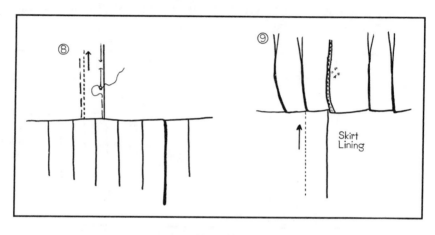

Sew snap(s) to overlap at waist as needed. Apply sealant or overcast any little places near waist seam that are exposed and might give you trouble later. Finish neck. Before you can sew the remainder of the waist seam, clip seam allowance just beyond zipper tape to stitches on overlap side. Due to the nature of the placket, it is impossible for your friend to precisely place the center front and the side seams in the pleated skirt when she checks the hem and arranges the pleats around the waist. Therefore, after you have finished the opening at the back of the dress, move the pleated skirt (only) slightly as required to fit the bodice. Pin and baste in position. Next, pin and baste lining to the bodice/skirt unit at waistline. Machine-stitch. Press seam upward beyond clip. Overcast seam.

SEPARATE SKIRTS AND TROUSERS

#14 SEPARATE SKIRT

For the all-around pleated skirt follow the skirt and placket directions suggested for the dress with a pleated skirt, except that the zipper stops at the waistline. For most other skirts arrange the skirt layers as for a dress described in #7 and prepare the placket for the zipper. For all skirts read Lining Yardage in ch. 4 regarding the strange behavior of belt colors. Follow the general directions for hems at the end of this chapter.

#15 TROUSERS

Handle just as for any partially connected lining explained in ch. 7: sew the lining and then sew the chiffon, always using the appropriate seam finishes. Join at the waist and placket using the details in this chapter. Sew to the band as always, paying attention to Lining Yardage, ch. 4. Hem as you would a dress of the same length or as appropriate.

HEMS

The finishing touch for your sheer garment is the hem that hangs perfectly. Except for such designs as those cut with handkerchief points or deliberately high in front, the skirt hem should hang evenly all around.

Some purists say the hand-rolled hem is the only one fine enough for chiffon. Don't believe it. If you go to all that trouble for a street length dress there is just a chance that due to its shorter length your friends will notice and admire your work. What about the floor-length gown? You probably wear it after dark in artificial light which may be flatteringly dim. You may be on a crowded dance floor or seated with your feet beneath a table. In such situations you can scarcely seen see the hem. How many times have you had a woman stoop over and pick up the hem of your skirt to examine it? Probably never.

You have three criteria for the chiffon hem. It must look pretty from the right side, it must hang evenly and it must not fray out.

Hems in garments made from other sheers follow the same rules. For the more opaque sheers, however, you have just a little bit of leeway. You can have a deeper hem if the little easing doesn't show from the right side. For that, see #17, Method II. Otherwise, these suggestions for sheer hems apply to all.

A word of caution: when you trim the bottom of the skirt make the cuts smooth and even -- little jagged places may show through the fine cloth.

#16 MARK THE HEM

Street-Length Put on the finished garment, belt it if necessary, wear the correct shoes and underwear and have your friend mark the finished length. Replace the pins with hand basting. This is the point of departure. Unless you plan some unusual skirt treatment, always add to this length; to cut off would make the dress too short.

Long Gown Put on the finished sheer garment, belt it if necessary and step into shoes with the correct heel height. Have your friend put pins where the sheer touches the floor. She smooths down the skirt and presses her thumbnail against the floor through the sheer. She does not stretch the cloth nor let it balloon out. Her thumbnail marks the spot for the pin. Pins should be no farther apart than 4 in. Remove the dress carefully so you won't lose the pins, and replace with hand basting -- hand basting because at this stage it is the most accurate method. Later you may replace with machine basting if required by stitching right next to the handwork.

A floor-length dress doesn't actually touch the floor. When the hem is marked you probably stand very erect. If you slump even a little it will drag the floor inviting the next passerby in a crowded room to step on it; or you can step on it yourself. The only exception to this is if you will be on a greatly elevated stage. The hem of the long skirt should escape the floor by at least 1/2 in.

#17 NARROW HEM FOR STREET-LENGTH DRESS

Method I (fig. 8-12)   Machine baste next to hand-basted mark that indicates the bottom of hem. **1.** Turn skirt wrong side up and place newsprint under your fabric. Using your presser foot as a guide, machine-baste 1/8 in. away -- into hem area --through sheer and paper. With your rotary cutter trim 1/8 in. beyond machine basting. **2.** With skirt still wrong side up press little strip of sheer up against the wrong side of skirt while you rest your iron on narrow band of paper and push against the machine basting. This forces all the sheer to turn up. It's optional if

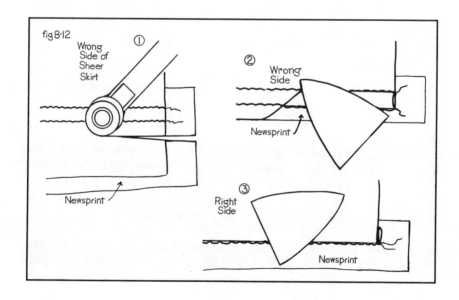

you machine baste through sheer and paper to hold in place. **3.** Turn skirt over to right side; paper is again underneath. Turn hem again toward wrong side, pressing on machine basting that marks finished hem length. You may now stitch in hem on the machine from the right side going through paper or remove last basting, tear paper away and hem by hand. Always remove necessary basting before you tear paper away. After that, remove original mark of finished length as in 6-11, step 5.

You may make this hem a little wider if you wish; simply substitute 1/4 in. (or whatever narrow width you need) for each 1/8 in. you read above.

Method II (fig. 8-13) A similar way to make the narrow hem is used by Patricia Marrow who is a charter member of MASS, is a certified instructor of their method and has a masters design certificate. Having retired from her own sewing school, she now has The Paris Connection -- *and* makes bridal gowns, as well. Her favorite method may suit your needs better because it doesn't use paper.

1. Mark finished hemline. Press toward the wrong side 1/8 in. below marked hem. **2.** If area needs stabilizing, stitch again using regular stitches 1/8 in. beyond pressed turn-up. If you need to ease in a bit of cloth because of curve, you may "stay stitch plus" -- pack more cloth per stitch by holding your finger behind presser foot, forcing the issue. Trim the excess fabric by cutting close to staystitching; take care not to cut one. **3.** Turn up on marked hem; press if you need an assist to position and stitch near first pressed fold. This makes a neat narrow hem.

This hem may be made wider, too

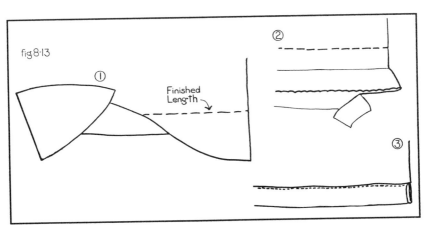

#18 HEM FOR LONG GOWN (fig. 8-14)

Here is one example of using the aforementioned floor- length hem mark. Suppose you want a hem that measures 1/4 in. **1.** Machine-baste 1/2 in. above floor mark. Cut cloth away on original hand basting (the floor mark). **2. Turn** this new raw edge up to touch machine-basted marks. Baste to hold if you like. **3.** Turn up again, this time on machine-basted mark. Put in hem by hand with running stitch or your favorite method.

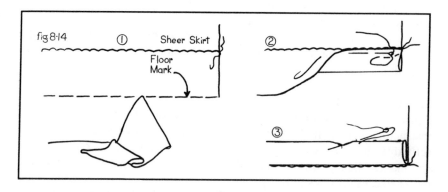

#19 HEMS FOR UNDERSKIRTS AND LINING (fig. 8-15)

Sew hem in sheer garment. Hang it on a suit hanger and suspend it from a doorway so that you can situate yourself at eye level to the hem. Shake hems out, arrange so they hang correctly and while you sit on something the right height, put pins in underskirt at edge of sheer hem where it extends below. Remove from the hanger and replace pins with hand basting in the underskirt layer only. When you've finished hemming this second layer of skirt, it should be 3/8 in. shorter than the sheer skirt. Use the thread marker as a guide and cut and hem accordingly. You may put this hem by hand or machine.

After the underskirt hem has been put in, repeat the procedure for the lining skirt. It, in turn, is about 3/8 in. shorter than the underskirt. If there is no underskirt, the lining is then 3/8 in. shorter than the sheer.

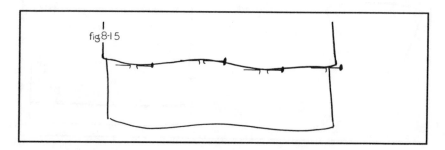

When an underskirt or lining hangs below the dress hem it completely shatters the illusion of beauty. That's bad enough. But should either be a different color than the sheer skirt, the ruination is complete. Although the under layers are vital to the performance of the outer garment, they are, after all, only supporting players that allow the sheer to be the star.

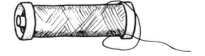

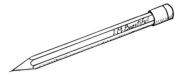

9

ALTERNATIVES

There are dozens of way of handling sheers not mentioned earlier. However, you can have the most fun with chiffon because it is so sheer. This chapter presents ideas that allow you to veer away from the traditional chiffon look. Silk chiffon is so lovely and expensive you probably wouldn't dream of using it for these new suggestions except for one or two of them. But a synthetic with its usually more modest price opens the door to all manner of innovations. However, this chapter only scratches the surface. Don't stop with just these ideas -- spread your wings and do something new and exciting. Have fun with sheer sewing.

Are you ready? Surely you've read ch. 5 and its companions chs. 4 and 6! If you're impatient you probably skipped right to these pages. After deciding what you want to make, better give those chapters a quick reading even if you plan to make something that's very informal. Those time-tested methods save headaches in the long run.

INFORMAL

Let's look at three very informal uses of chiffon. Even the young beginner can make #1 and #10.

#1 BRIEF SKIRT (fig. 9-1)

Wear this very simple unlined sheer skirt over leotards for school, at-home or exercise class. It depends on what is acceptable in your community. Boldly flowered chiffon is the cloth choice of most teens. The pull-on style is the easiest to make and wear. Although the length is a matter of the current fashion in the community, about 15 in. is the maximum.

Get Ready If the cloth is 60 in. wide you need buy only 1/2 yd., but because you can usually find a brilliant pattern in only 44 in. width, the example is geared accordingly.

147

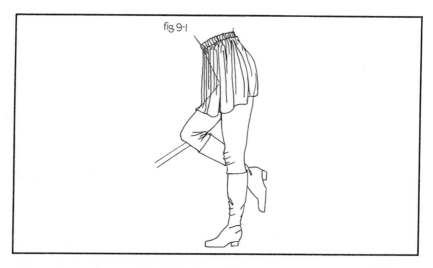

fig. 9-1

Buy twice the finished length plus about 3 or 3 1/2 in. if the fabric has been torn. If it hasn't, buy a little more and pull a thread to even it after you get home. Have the salesperson tear the chiffon when you buy it. After you've prepared the fabric as suggested in ch. 5, tear the fabric crosswise to separate in two equal pieces. Trim off selvages.

Serger Method (fig. 9-2) **1.** Serge the sides together (the ones from which you trimmed the selvages) to form a large tube. Serge the single layer of cloth around the top to finish raw edge. **2.** Measure width of elastic, add 3/8 in. and fold down top that amount. Machine-stitch down middle of serged stitches leaving open a space at start and finish wide enough to admit elastic.

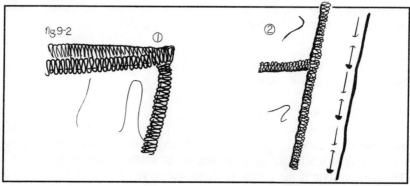

fig. 9-2

3. Measure your waist, add about 1 in. and cut elastic that length (or follow directions on elastic package). Thread elastic in casing. Overlap ends and sew together. You may close the opening you left for elastic by machine or hand-stitching. Try on and check length. **4.** Adjust your serger as required and make a rolled hem at the bottom edge.

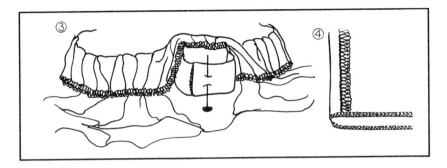

If you need to press serging before you sew casing, use vinegar water solution, ch. 5. It looks neater if you press side seams to one side.

Sewing Machine Method You will find ch. 6 helpful. Sew side seams together in French seams making a large tube. For waist casing for elastic, turn down 1/4 in. at top. Measure elastic, add 1/4 in. and turn down top again that amount. Or follow steps 1 and 2, fig. 8-12, except substitute 1/4 in. for 1/8 in. and make casing deep enough to accommodate the wide waist elastic. Leave space to admit elastic as above, step 3, and handle elastic the same. Try on skirt and check length. Apply machine rolled hem, fig. 6-8, or simple narrow machine hem, fig. 8-12.

#2 LOUNGER (fig. 9-3)

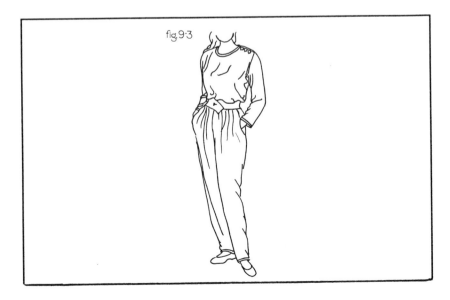

fig. 9-3

The only reason you mount chiffon on knit and sew with your serger is because the knit feels so good against the skin. Of course, chiffon won't stretch but if you remember this important fact, you'll be all right. Follow the same general ideas for colors you see in other paragraphs in this and other chapters. Although when you put the two fabrics together the knit seems to grow, the results are great for those special at-home affairs. You want to appear just lounging around watching television in ordinary clothes -- which just happen to be very subtly gorgeous. True, these won't stand rough wear but they're not supposed to.

Get Ready Cut out the sheer according to instructions in ch. 5. Cut out the knit as usual. Be sure you can pull on trousers without stretching the cloth -- the chiffon has no give. Along the same line, if the garment has a simple neck finish, such as ribbing, that requires you to stretch it to pull over your head, you need to open the shoulder seam to make a placket. Although you could install a zipper, the example shows the changes necessary for buttons. Follow the suggestions in this chapter in #6 and #7 for mounting the chiffon to another cloth. Stitch the right shoulder seam as usual but leave the left shoulder open 4 1/4 in. from neck stitches. (Test to see if this is large enough for your head.)

Change Pattern (fig. 9-4) The back neck facing is all right the way it is. The front neck facing needs an extension for buttonhole reinforcement. If your pattern envelope doesn't have facing patterns, refer to 5-1 but cut only 1 1/2 in. deep. Extend left front facing shoulder seam (and cutting line) from neck stitches twice the shoulder opening plus 1 in. In this example that's 9 1/2 in. From shoulder seam measure down enough to accommodate the buttons; we use 1 1/2 in. Extension will fold back on itself. (Or cut 1/2 length and use iron-on interfacing.)

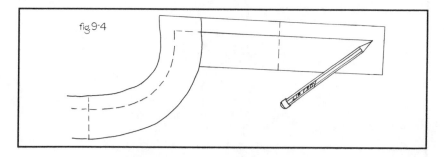

fig 9-4

Cut a pattern for patch (the underlap) on which you will sew buttons. It is also twice the width needed from the neck stitches plus 1 in., in our case 9 1/2 in. Patch also folds in half.

Sew New Neck (9-5) Cut out facings and patch. Sew *right* shoulder seam of facings together. Serge around them except for actual neck edges. Fold patch over and then serge around the three sides.

The following neck stitching is better if done with regular sewing machine stitches. **1.** Place patch on left back shoulder about 3/16 in. from neck seam. With everything else out of the way, pin to back. Place facing on top and pin all around neck. **2.** Fold front left buttonhole extension over on itself to neck seam and, keeping everything else out of the way, pin to shoulder seam. Turn unit over so you can see termination of previous shoulder stitching. Sew shoulder/neck seam, pulling out pins as you come to them.

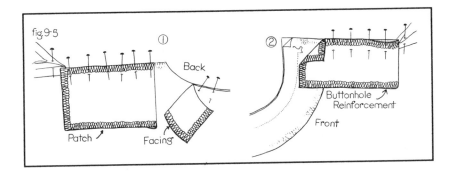

3. Trim off corners and neck seam as required by your pattern and turn facings to inside. **4.** Bring patch toward front. Topstitch according to style of garment. Make buttonholes in front going through chiffon, knit and reinforcement following tips in 7-13. Sew buttons on patch. You can put a bar-tack across shoulder seam at opening to strengthen.

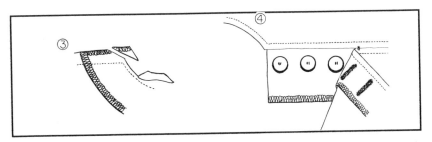

CHIFFON AND FRIENDS

#3 TWIN PRINTS

Motomachi Street in Yokohama is an international shopping area where, due to its proximity to that Japanese port, one finds delights from all over the world. One day a strolling tourist spied a memorable dress in a fashionable shop window that made a lasting impression on her. The skirt, a sophisticated chiffon print, was spread out dramatically to reveal that its free-hanging lining was made from the matching print in crepe. Where was this beauty created -- Italy? Paris? No one knows, but the visitor will long remember her first exposure to this creative use of these companions.

Twin prints -- one of chiffon and the other in an opaque fabric -- are fun to work with and give you plenty of latitude for experimentation. You can sew sleeves and bodice from the sheer while you make the skirt from the opaque; make a dress from opaque fabric and a loose coat from the sheer, to name but two ideas.

If you have shopped very much for these look-alikes you know how hard it is to find what you want; so often what is available is not to your taste. After a long search you finally find a fabric design you really like only to learn that the matching print was sold out days before. You tromp from store to store becoming more discouraged with each step.

Here's a solution that may work for you: find a fabric design in chiffon which pleases you greatly. Use its background color for lining and mount the chiffon for the opaque sections while you use the chiffon as it is for the sheer areas. Proceed to sew the garment(s) using the appropriate techniques for each part.

#4 PLEATED CHIFFON

Machine pleating and chiffon seem to be made for each other and this happy marriage enables you to turn out professional looking garments. Sometimes you can buy both pleated and matching unpleated fabric to sew in almost unending combinations. There are many varieties of pleats to choose from -- sunburst, knife-pleats, regular pleats of all widths, and novelties. You can even send off your polyester to be pleated to your liking. See Additional Information. This service frees you from relying on the selection in the store -- or no selection at all. You can also have matching fabric, such as taffeta, pleated. From the portion of a sleeve to an entire shift, pleats enable you to produce an expensive looking garment that does not advertise you made it at home.

#5 MAKE A BORDER PRINT

You can use this on any plain sheer.

When you buy a border print you are at the mercy of the design. You must place it so it falls near a central seam, forms an edge on a straight-cut collar, follows the hem or use in some other restrictive fashion. There's an alternative if you are artistic (which of course you are). Apply the design where you want it either by fabric painting or fabric dying.

Let's assume you want to "paint" a border on otherwise plain fabric near the hem of a flared skirt. Using a very simple dress pattern with few distracting details, cut out the garment in the synthetic fabric. Sew the skirt together using your muslin trial to tell you precisely where the hem turn-up will be. Proceed with the decorating and place the design exactly where you want it. You should do the coloring business before you make the entire garment; in case of a mishap no great amount of money or labor is lost.

Of course, this takes planning to make the design come out correctly so the start and finish look continuous. But there is a saving grace: since people can't look at all parts of the design at once, you can cheat a bit here and there, perhaps leave out one little part or add a little extra somewhere to make the join unnoticeable. You will work it out on paper, first, of course.

You can position a design anywhere on the dress you please. Place bold, stylized flowers irregularly on the skirt front, add a border to the bottom of loose sleeves or follow an interesting neckline to name but a few. What you produce will be an original, one of a kind.

It is beyond the scope of this book to instruct you how to execute these procedures. You probably already have some experience with this type work and have a good idea where you can use it on your sheer garment. After reading the instructions that come with the equipment, you will try them out on scraps of your fabric to test how its color changes the applied color. Just be sure to use a product that can stand up to the type care you must give it, whether it's washing or dry cleaning. If at all possible, try to give shading to designs. More than any other technique, this gives authority to your work. Remember to fix for permanency if required.

#6 MOUNTING FOR BEAUTY

By this time you know that mounting is a method whereby each piece of fashion fabric is sewn to an exactly matching piece of lining and thereafter handled as a single layer of cloth. When working with chiffon this technique is useful when you wish to produce a completely different color scheme from a chiffon print, perhaps one more suitable for your complexion. Virtually any fairly simple dress or suit pattern may be used as long as the lining fabric is quite soft and flexible.

Shopping   Choose a very sheer chiffon print that has plenty of light-colored areas. Experiment while you are in the store by laying it over various colors of lining until you find the result that pleases you. Notice how drastically the lining colors change the appearance of the chiffon. Again, the sheerer the chiffon, the more interesting the result. You may want to play around with different colors behind the sheer while you are in the quiet of your home undistracted by people or noise.

Yardage for both chiffon and lining is figured as described in ch. 4 except that if you use an unusual color for the lining, such as green, you must decide whether or not to line the sleeves. If you do not, the dress may look as if it were made from one fabric and the sleeves from another. Consider lining the sleeves with a layer of chiffon the same color as the lining. You may end up lining the sleeves, too. Whatever your decision, try it out in the store. Almost every major pattern piece needed for the garment will be needed for both layers, common sense being your guide. You may find it more comfortable if you make the back neck facing from fine cotton/poly broadcloth that matches. You can interface with that fabric, too, or eliminate it altogether -- you must judge for yourself if there's enough body.

Prep and Cut Prepare, cut and label the fabrics as for any other chiffon garment. Remember, no need to mark on chiffon because the lining carries the marks. Place a cut-out piece of lining face up on the table. (The other side has the marks, if any.) On top of it place and pin its matching piece of chiffon. Hand-baste the two together about 1/2 in. from all edges. Baste down the centers of any darts to hold the layers together when you stitch on the machine. Baste near center front, etc.

Pleats Does your garment have pleats? Baste near fold line of any pleat. Turn garment wrong side out and take little back-stitches about 1/4 in. apart on the marked fold line sending the needle through both lining and chiffon. See 7-6, step 4. Work from left to right so you see the longer "dashes" of thread on the inside of the dress and the small "dots" on the outside. The thread should be very fine, non- glossy and an exact match. Do not draw the threads so tightly as to make little dents on the right side of the skirt. To crease the fold that points on the outside, turn the garment right side out and fold exactly on the stitchline; the lining sides touch. Hand-baste as you work the length of the pleat. Press, using the vinegar-water solution but stop short of the hem area which you finish when the hem has been put in. To crease the underpleat, fold the chiffon sides together and proceed as above.

When you are working with a busy print or will wear the dress under artificial light, the backstitches that hold the two layers together probably won't show. However, when you want your plain-colored chiffon to withstand the *closest* scrutiny in any light, the answer is to ravel out some of the chiffon and use that for the thread. Although such thread is fine almost to the point of invisibility and twists around itself, it's perfect for the job because it meets all the requirements mentioned above. Use a needle threader, pull the strand half way through the needle so you can use it double and cut the strand to release the needle threader. Sew where there is plenty of strong light and work slowly. Pull the strands through each time leaving no loops on the right side. Check the right side occasionally to see if it looks all right. On the finished dress you cannot see these little stitches even in strongest daylight but they hold the lining against the chiffon.

If the backstitches of regular threads show on the right side but this does not bother you, or your eyes won't allow you to do the chiffon/thread business, be satisfied with the results of the regular thread. After all, just so much perfection is required.

Hem When you are ready to hem, put the garment on a coat hanger and pin through both layers above where you will sew the hem. Remove from the hangar and substitute hand-basting for the pins. Now you're ready to have your friend mark the length. There's no need for a deep hem but you should apply seam tape to the raw edge to avoid bulk. Sew hem in by hand sending the needle through only the lining layer and then the tape. Remove the skirt basting and press the pleats near the hem. Press the hem edge just a little -- only enough to achieve the soft look you want.

#7 TWO LAYERS OF CHIFFON

When you make unmounted chiffon in a tailored design, it becomes softened and dressy, perfect for the woman who feels foolish in flowing garments, but wants enhancement for special occasions. What follows is a most intriguing method, usually for the street-length dress, that is so versatile it is equally at home with the tailored dress or that beautifully cut special design. The basic procedure is simple; the results are quite extraordinary. Garments made this way have tantalizing, elusive shadows caused by the interplay of colors. Not a traditional chiffon look, this system produces a new effect and chiffon is the instrument. The subtle unmatched elegance of such a garment makes it suitable for such rarified occasions as:

Mother of The Bride
The Reception For the Ambassador
Tea With the President's Wife

This method relies heavily on correct fit and a flattering style. If you have a favorite dress that fits well and brings you many complements, now is the time to use the pattern again. Or use any pattern that is fairly simple, not tightly fitted and with few if any gathers -- which, unless you are quite thin, will make you look heavy. However, folds, pleats and tucks which are fairly flat create different planes and surfaces that display mysterious shadows.

The Rehearsal Make the dress first in muslin as directed in ch. 1 if it's a new pattern. Next, consider what your activities will be during your special occasion. If you will be standing or moving around in a certain way (such as swinging your arms to christen a ship) try out these movements in front of a full-length mirror while you wear the muslin trial dress. Will you be seated most of the time? Seat yourself in front of a big mirror to see if the muslin dress looks pretty. You want no gaps or puffs; the dress that looks great while you stand erect may not pass the test while you sit relaxed. Few of us can maintain perfect posture very long. When you are satisfied with the fit and have calculated the yardage as explained in ch. 4, you are ready to go shopping.

Shopping Probably no other field of sewing allows you to paint with cloth so fully. You are not shopping for one color of chiffon but two. The beauty of the dress lies in the subtle blending of the two colors of chiffon and the equally important interaction of their weaves against each other and the lining. Understand this: the more sheer the upper layer of chiffon, the easier the colors will blend. Or, put another way, if the upper layer is slightly opaque, the second layer must be a very strong color. You will have an exciting time in the fabric store experimenting with an almost unending combination of colors.

You will have immense success with clear pink over deep orange which produces an indescribable coral. Royal blue over sharp apple green produces a quiet shimmering turquoise. Here are some other combinations that look well together:

> Pink over yellow
> Yellow over orange
> Royal blue over sky blue, turquoise, aqua or orange
> Royal blue over most strong colors
> Dark brown over most strong colors
> Black over brown or over most strong rich colors

But don't stop there. Try any combinations that come to mind. Remember, the sheerness of the top layer of chiffon can affect the resulting color.

Keep in mind that the lining, which must be very flexible, can bring the two colors to their greatest potential. Eggshell or a palest pink work well because you do not line the sleeves. Even if your skin is dark, however, these are still good lining colors. (Read the latter part of ch. 4 under Color.) While in the store you must work with three layers of cloth during this color testing period. It helps if you have a big square of the lining you can carry to eliminate one bolt of cloth.

Lighting The next thing to consider is the lighting. Try the two colors plus the lining in the light conditions of your special occasion. Fluorescent light is no problem. You're in it at the store. If it will be incandescent light, as most of us use in our living rooms, you will not likely find it in the fabric shop display room. They may have such lighting in the storeroom which they would allow you to use. Otherwise, better take some samples home to test in the proper lighting conditions. This is important. One woman was quite dismayed to learn that the dress made in emerald green over intense sky blue that looked a lovely greenish blue in the daytime, appeared just plain green at night under incandescent light. Although not all colors and fibers react this way, some do. Try out your color combinations in the correct lighting situation to make sure you're not wasting your time and money.

This exciting shopping expedition can be ruined if you attempt to do it when the store is crowded with other customers. By planning such exacting buying during the slack time, the appreciation of the store manager and his assistants will be reflected by their cooperation. (Refer to the last paragraph of ch. 4.)

Prep and Cut Prepare and cut the fabrics as described in ch. 5, but mark only the lining. Lay a cut-out piece of lining face up on a large table and examine it carefully for any threads or snips of cloth. They will show up later and, short of ripping the dress apart, you will be unable to remove them. Next, cut out the under layer of chiffon and place the appropriate piece of it carefully on top of the lining, matching the centers, etc. Examine this piece, too, for threads and the like. Pin and then baste the two layers together by hand in the seam allowance. Next, cut out the top layer of chiffon and place it on top of the other layers already joined, check for threads and then baste to the other two.

Do not put markings on either piece of chiffon except to indicate a patch pocket location, and that indication goes only on the top layer.

You will notice that no matter how carefully you cut out, one piece or the other of chiffon will be a little larger here and there. After you have basted them together, simply trim carefully so any chiffon that extends beyond the lining is eliminated. We're assuming that the lining is cut with less deviation from the pattern cutting-line.

DON'T attempt to cut out the two layers of chiffon at the same time. It is more difficult and certainly more time-consuming than to cut them one at a time. Not only would you have to fiddle with two layers of wiggly cloth but you could not achieve the accuracy you need for true straight of grain. That is of prime importance because without it the dress would not hang perfectly as a unit. This is essential with mounted layers.

Sewing Suggestions Construct the dress as if it were one piece of fabric in the usual fashion except for the special situations mentioned in MOUNTING FOR BEAUTY. Again, you may want to substitute cotton for the back neck facing -- one always gets hot and excited during an important occasion.   Also, consider eliminating the interfacing.   It's possible the special places will now have enough body; stiffness is out of order. Buttons can be covered quite satisfactorily professionally if you pin the three layers of cloth together and explain which is right side up. Don't let the color of the button foundation discolor the end product.

This most impressive creation is the answer when you must avoid anything hinting at flashiness. People seldom recognize chiffon as the fabric but they are quick to appreciate the lovely soft effect.

Variations There are many variations of TWO LAYERS of CHIFFON construction. If you use lace as the under layer, test stiffness when you consider a pattern. Although the effect is somewhat different, it produces an interesting garment and is suitable for a coat, the dress with a bouffant skirt and others. Check to see of you need to use two layers of chiffon to counteract the color density of the lining cloth. The skirt layers need not be sewn together and can hang separately. By using your imagination you will come up with many other variations.

#8 THE STAY-PUT BLOUSE
This concerns the blouse that you tuck in your skirt or trousers, not an over-blouse. Do you share the problem with the woman who must stand stock-still so that her top doesn't pull out making her look sloppy instead of casual? If so, this section may solve your problem.

Almost every blouse design on any particular woman looks its best and flatters the wearer the most when it falls over the skirt band a particular amount -- not more, not less. Have you ever put on your suit skirt and tuck-in blouse and then tugged at the blouse a little to allow it to fall over the skirt just a certain amount to look more relaxed, less precisely placed? People with slim hips do this.

Perhaps you lean another direction. After donning your skirt and blouse you comb your hair. Then you reach up under your skirt to tug your blouse down. You know instinctively what look is most flattering to you. To allow yourself to move naturally while you wear the outfit, you'd better do something to keep everything in place so you won't have to fiddle with your clothes as you go about your activities.
These paragraphs are for the woman who knows she looks her best when her blouse has only a modest amount of ease. We have two

examples. Although the results are the same, with the first you have the help of a friend. (Read the first one even if you must work alone.) You may think as you read that there will be no blousing at all. However, there is always some because the strap must be loose enough for comfort.

The versatile blouse (fig. 9-6) with tucks that go from shoulder yoke to hem, made from any soft cloth from finest crepe to chiffon, is

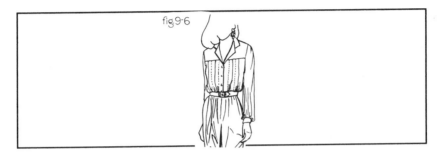

fig 9-6

suitable to wear with trousers or skirt. You can adapt this system to the blouse without a yoke if you line it from shoulder to hem with a soft lining of an appropriate color -- flesh-color, blouse-color or whatever is correct.

When You Have Help (fig. 9-7) Don the altered trial muslin shift which represents the lining. See 3-6. **1.** Have your friend tie a string around your waist and arrange gathers; there is no blousing. With the string in place, mark above it with the felt-tipped pen. On side seam mark 2 in. below wide hip level the approximate crotch depth. **2.** Put on the muslin blouse. Match center fronts, side seams and center back. Pin the yoke

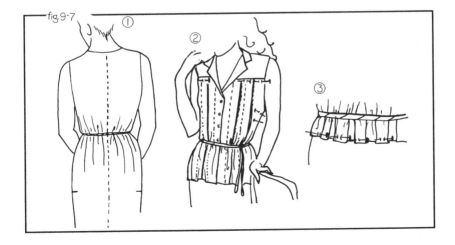

fig 9-7

seamline as in 3-6, steps 4 and 5. Tie another string around blouse waist. Arrange gathers to flatter your figure and pin every 2 in. around waist. **3.** Cut off muslin blouse so it extends 2 in. below the string. Pin upper muslin to lining muslin so gathers at this dropped position are in the same location as held by string. Remove pins at waist.

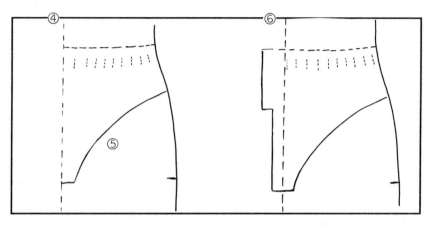

Remove pinned-together muslin garments carefully. Mark each pin location with the pen on the blouse muslin. Do not unpin. **4.** With the aid of transfer paper and the wheel, mark each pin location on lining. **5.** Draw a curving line on back lining from side seam something like a high-cut panty-line as shown. **6.** Repeat for the front. (Because the blouse opens down the front, the strap must fasten low at wide hip level so it will pass over the hips easily; you will step into the blouse to put it on.) Follow 3-6, steps 6, 7, 8 and 9, to mark yoke cutting line on lining.

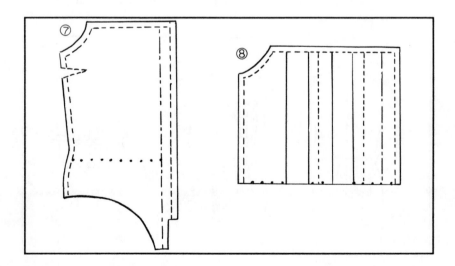

Transfer all changes to facsimiles. **7.** Cut away lining pattern below curving line. Front lining pattern will look something like the illustration. **8.** Cut blouse pattern 2 in. below waist. Front blouse pattern will look something like the illustration.

When You Work Alone (fig. 9-8) Don the altered shift. **1.** Tie a string around your waist and arrange the gathers attractively. Draw above string with felt-tipped pen. Leave string in place. With the pen mark what you judge to be a good shape for bottom of lining as shown. Front must be placed low so when you step into the blouse it will pass easily over your hips, but not so low you can't undo fasteners with ease. **2.** Put on the blouse muslin and match center fronts and side seams. As best you can, pin the yoke to lining muslin as in 3-6, steps 4 and 5. Tie a string around your waist and arrange gathers attractively. Using the felt-tipped pen, mark just above string. Pin gathers in place all around waist just below string. Catch lining, too, with pins. **3.** Carefully remove pinned-together garments. Mark each pin location with the pen on blouse muslin. Don't remove pins. Using transfer paper and wheel, mark these locations on lining. Also, following 3-6, steps 6, 7, 8 and 9, make cutting line for yoke on lining. Transfer all changes and notations to lining and blouse facsimiles.

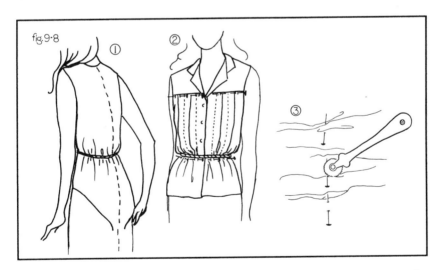

fig. 9-8

4. On lining pattern measure down from waistline 2 in. Move the pin marks straight down to this dropped line and indicate their location. Cut away pattern below curved line for strap. **5.** On blouse pattern measure down 2 in. from waist and mark. Move pin locations straight down to dropped mark. Cut away pattern below this new bottom line. Your new front patterns will look the same as if you have help.

Whether you work alone or have help you are ready to complete the pattern.   On the blouse pattern erase the unneeded waistline indication. A misplaced mark would show through the delicate cloth.

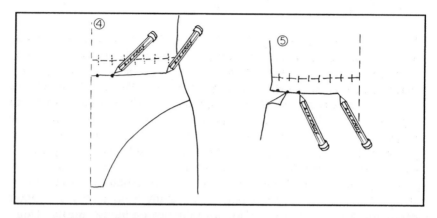

Strap Pattern This extension of the center back is a strap, slightly shaped at the connecting end and tapering to 2 1/2 in. or 3 in. wide. It passes between the legs where it fastens low in front with buttons or grippers. You may cut it as an extension of your lining fabric, but piecing on with matching poly/cotton is better. The seam, being so low in the back, will not cause a ridge to show through even the tightest skirt. Years ago girls' gym shirts were made this way. No matter how strenuous the sport, the blouse couldn't come out.   The same idea is used today for the body stocking except this version is not as fitted and doesn't require a knit fabric.

Working with the muslin lining, cut the strap the length you think will be correct plus 3 or 4 in. Try on and raise your arms -- you want it to be rather snug but not bind. (This is why you always have some blousing.)

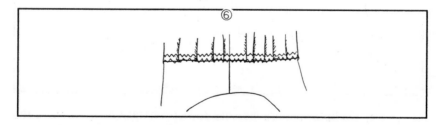

Sew the Blouse Sew the body of the blouse according to the general directions in ch. 7 under YOKES. To connect the bottom of this blouse to the lining, match side seams and center back and then the pin marks of the fashion fabric to those on the lining. Pin the little pleats in place and then zigzag over the raw edge of the blouse. **6.** Zigzag again just above for a very flat, smooth appearance over the hips and abdomen. See illustration number 6 in the group above.

Sew the Lower Regions (fig. 9-9) **1.** After you have calculated the correct comfortable length, add about 3 in. at the end for reinforcement for the buttonholes. **2.** Sew the strap to back lining, right sides together, taking a 1/2 in. seam.

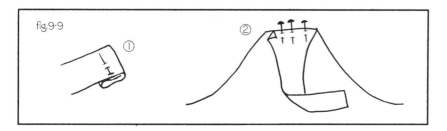

3. Sew the low front lining together for 2 1/2 in. Clip to seam to accommodate front blouse closure. Test to see if you can draw it on over the hips with ease. Reinforce the low front lining to handle the buttons by cutting a patch of poly/cotton the width of the strap and 3 in. deep. Fold in half and overcast the edges. Sew in place on the inside with regular stitches. Turn lining 1/2 in. toward the inside and zigzag over raw edge (except for center front). Strap connection folds up, too. **4.** Zigzag sides of strap to finish and put buttonholes in end. Sew buttons to front.

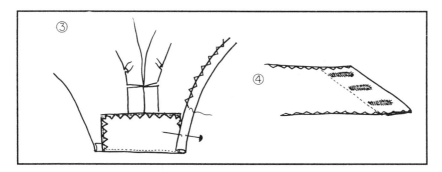

Instead of sewing buttons below waistline, sew one hook and thread eye about 1 in. below waist. **5.** You may cut away front overlap below hook down to low seam of lining and finish with an over-edge stitch. The serger is perfect for this. This insures a flat finish and being under the skirt, it will never be seen. You can put a bar-tack across seam.

Once you know just how high to cut the lining on the side seams and how long and wide to make the strap, you will want to use this method often. You have none of those restrictions on movement fearing you'll pull out your shirt or blouse. You look tidy without fussing with your clothes.

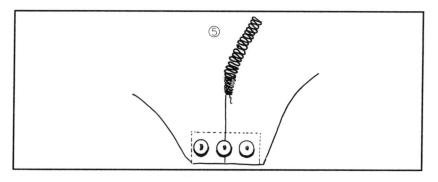

#9 CIRCLE RUFFLE (fig. 9-10)

The ruffle made from a circle, besides using fabric most efficiently, produces a lovely fluted edge. The inner circle wants to lie flat in a curve and you force it into a straight line. All the rest of the cloth in the circle has to ripple to allow the inner circle to assume this new shape. Try encasing fishing line in the zigzag stitches at the outer edge of an organza circle to produce a stiff edge that looks completely professional. Although it seems that you could use a strip of bias and achieve the same results, you can't. The look is different and not as elegant.

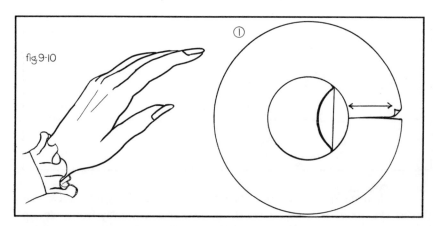

fig 9-10

The application at the wrist of a plain fitted sleeve is used in the example although there are many other uses. Adjust the measurements to suit your situation. Cut sleeve slightly longer than the finished length.

1. The outside circle diameter should not be less than 7 in. so set your compass with a radius of 3 1/2 in. Keep the point in the same spot and reset the radius for 1 1/2 in. for the inner circle. Slash mark should be on the straight of grain. Discard the inner circle.

2. Set the machine to sew the very fine zigzag to finish the edge or use the serger to make a rolled edge. For a wrist you need only one circle ruffle of this size. **3.** Immediately before you apply, trim sleeve so it measures 3/16 in. longer than this finish requires (which you determine when making the muslin trial). Pin the ruffle to outside of sleeve edge to test the length. Cut to size. Join ends of the ruffle on the wrong side with the very fine zigzag rolled edge. **4.** Pin ruffle to the right side of sleeve, raw edges even and machine-stitch a narrow seam with the very fine stitch. Repeat, using the very fine zigzag causing a rolled hem. Or make the rolled edge/seam on serger in one step.

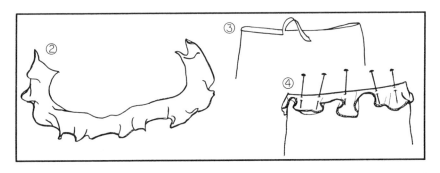

Don't press but baste the tiny seam, if any, against the inside of sleeve. This is great to do on the serger.

#10 BALLET PRACTICE SKIRT (fig. 9-11)

Another use for the circle ruffle is the brief skirt the ballet dancer ties around her waist over her leotard for practice. Make this from plain colored chiffon. The new sewer can even make this to give to a friend. Measure your waist and subtract 1/2 in. Decide the length you want the skirt in front and jot both these in your notebook. Divide new waist measurement by pi (3.14) to find the diameter. Divide this by 2 to get the radius and set your compass to this size between point and pencil lead. **1.** Draw this size circle on paper. Draw a line through the circle to indicate the center front and center back. Measure out from rim the length of skirt you want and make a pencil mark. **2.** Using the same spot for center, draw bigger circle passing through the pencil mark. Use a pin, string and pencil if you lack a great big compass. **3.** With your pencil shape the skirt to be a little longer in back. Cut around outside edge.

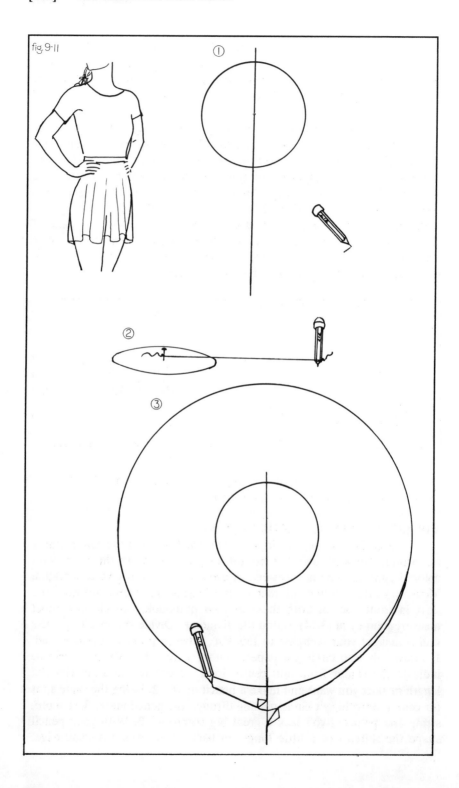

fig. 9-11

① ② ③

Cut on center back line. Cut out inner circle which you discard. This is the pattern.

Cut out skirt using tips in ch. 5, HOW TO CUT OUT, Pin On Pattern.

4. Serge the three sides indicated. Don't try to stretch cloth while stitching. **5.** Cut a length of satin or ribbon twice the width of finished band. For length cut waist measurement plus about 60 in. Fold over, even it's edges and press down it's length. **6.** Hold ends together and mark the middle with a press from the tip of the iron or a pencil mark.

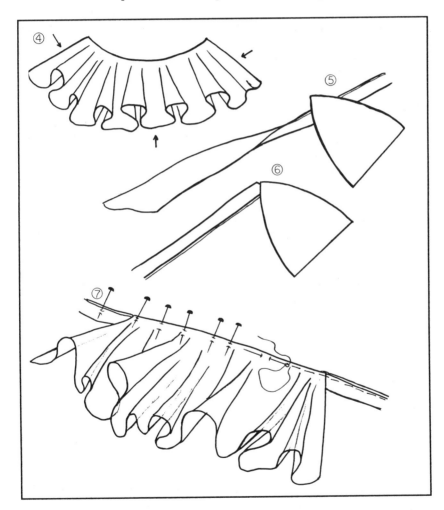

7. Match the center front mark of the skirt to the center mark of the band and pin together. Pin the rest of the skirt to band. (You may baste.) Being careful of the pins, tie around your waist to test-tie to decide your preferred length of ties. Trim if required. Start serging at the end of one tie and continue to end of other, removing pins as you come to them.

OTHER IDEAS

Chiffon On Wool

Ordinarily you don't line chiffon sleeves. But, read on.

One autumn when a traveler from the tropics visited cold damp Scotland she wondered if she would ever feel dry and warm again. Homes and public places weren't warm enough for her to wear her more dressy, filmy frocks. When she caught cold she cursed the miserable weather and dreamed of hot dry sand. She wondered if the Scottish women ever got tired of wearing woolens, lovely though they were. Why not cover the fine woolens with chiffon -- arms and all? It would be a slightly different look and they would be warm, as well.

Easy Casual "Camisole"

As a substitute for the camisole under a shirt or any casual top, wear a tubular knit with a drawstring at the top, or one of the tubes made of multiple rows of elastic stitches. Just be sure you have a really great figure with a flat diaphragm.

Trimming

There is no dearth of trimming ideas for chiffon. It's only hard to know where to stop listing them. Here are a few. You'll think of many more.

1. Cut narrow bias bands of soft satin-like material of the matching color and bind the neck, sleeves, etc.

2. Use very narrow, flexible grosgrain ribbon of a contrasting color to trim one special place.

3. Make an artificial flower of matching fabric or stiffened chiffon, add streamers made from bias tubes and pin it in back either at the base of a low V neck or at the waist.

4. Stitch three 1 in. tucks horizontally on sleeves, just above the skirt hem or around the hips.

5. Mount chiffon on doubleknit for the construction of a "casual" jacket. Hand-knit strips of matching yarn and insert along top of sleeve from shoulder-tip to wrist or down front from yoke to bottom. Or hand-knit entire sleeves. This is especially effective when done in a light color.

6. Make a band of vertical tucks and insert where needed. Not only are tucks and lace pretty in the upper sleeves, they also conceal.

7.   After working out your design on paper, back the sheer cloth appropriately and decorate with beads.

8. Go all out to make a tailored blouse using triple top- stitching on collar, cuffs, button front, yokes and pockets.

9. Make a jacket or blouse of chiffon scraps using the very fine stitch. Put the seams on the outside where you encourage them to ravel.

10. Use many, tiny, hand-painted buttons as the only trim.

11. Cover buttons in matching satin.

The key word for some of the above is "matching." If the color is off you will have a sale-rack garment.

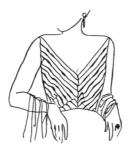

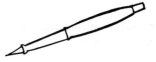

10

TIPS AND HINTS

Here's a potpourri of information to answer your lingering questions.

SNAPS AND HOOKS

#1 Years ago newspapers carried the big news that apartment house owners in the larger cities had started replacing operator-run elevators with self-service ones. How dismayed the women tenants were who lived alone! Were they worried about security? It's hard to imagine now, but in those days such women were relatively safe. No, their bewilderment was practical and personal. "Who in the world is going to fasten me up the back?" they cried. And well they might. Many of these operators had worked in the same building and had run the same elevator for years. They were practically family. When a lady tenant couldn't manage the fastener in back, the operator obliged.

Snaps are particularly hard to manage, but even if you're forced to knock on your neighbor's door for help, it may be worth it. This fine snap closure in a sheer unlined chiffon area allows a delicate appearance denied by the zipper. Be sure your friend, new-found or otherwise, has a strong light to work in when snapping you up, especially if your chiffon is a dark color.

#2 On the back bodice placket that's cloth bound, sew hooks in places of strain such as the shoulders and waist. Put on the muslin garment and ask your friend to watch (or work alone using two mirrors) and mark the places that need hooks while you touch your elbows together in front of yourself. In between, alternate snaps with hooks every inch or so. Mark these locations before you sew on any ornamental buttons.

#3 It is nearly impossible to cover tiny snaps with cloth. If you cannot buy colored or covered hooks and snaps to match your cloth, paint regular ones with nail polish before you sew them on. You can buy many weird shades at the variety stores -- even green, blue and the like. Those combined with your regular shades should do nicely. Place the snaps on a piece of paper and paint with the appropriate color, let dry thoroughly and re-coat as necessary. Hooks and snaps treated this way will not glitter metallically from between the folds of the closure.

CUFF WITH SNAPS

#4 Pin the cuff closed (fig. 10-1) so it fits comfortably when you slip one finger under it. **1.** With a pin or thread mark where the upper end reaches, remove the pin that holds the cuff together and take off the garment. Depending on the width of the cuff, sew two or three tiny snaps underneath the upper end of the cuff. Use the smaller half of the snap -- the one that has the bulb protruding on its right side. Position the snap, hide the knot under it and proceed to sew through each snap hole once, not going through to the right side. Start around again taking one stitch in the first hole. **2.** Then send the needle through to the right side.

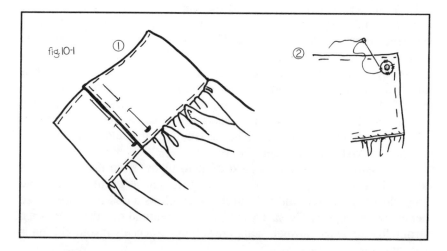

fig 10-1

3. Re-insert the needle very close to where the thread emerges, but peek to underside to see that it comes through the snap hole. Only a tiny dot of thread will show on the right side. Proceed round the snap in this manner. Then sew on each snap the same way. The propose is to hold the snap and the cuff facing out of sight without top stitching. The appearance is quite neat from the right side -- only four tiny dots show for each snap and they are almost unnoticeable. **4.** Lap the cuff according to the marker. Send a pin down through the hole of each snap you have sewn on. Lift the upper cuff just a bit and put a dot next to the spot where the pin pierces the under-cuff. Separate the cuff ends. **5.** Push a pin through the hole in the center of the under half of the snap and send the pin point into the dot. This holds the snap firmly in place while you sew it on in the ordinary way. Repeat for all snaps on the under-cuff.

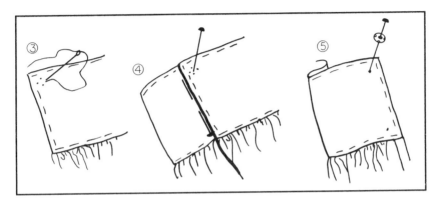

BUTTONS

#5 Tiny covered buttons of 1/4 in. are beyond compare when you want ornamental buttons to enhance a snap closure. To preserve the true color of the sheer, use two layers of lining together plus one or two of sheer for covering the buttons. This prevents a metallic gray from discoloring the finished work. Sew about 1/2 in. apart.

#6 Ornamental buttons, such as those above, are just for show. Decide how close together you want the buttons (pearls, etc.). Thread two needles with strong, fine thread that matches the sheer, usually chiffon. Figure 10-2, step **1.** At the neck sew on a tiny hook, colored to match the

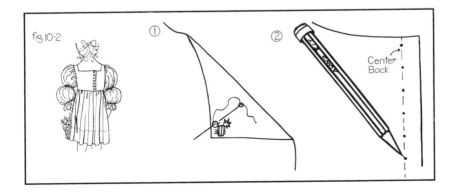

cloth, on the wrong side of the upper placket. As you have several layers of chiffon in that spot, sew through most of the layers for each hole. Then go through to the right side once for each hole and the shank. Secure the thread and cut it off. Lay that threaded needle aside. **2.** Place your first button immediately below this first hook. Starting at that point on the right side, put a little pencil mark (or other) on the center line every place you want a button. Continue marking the placket to the waist or bottom.

3. Pick up the other threaded needle and pierce the underside so the point of the needle comes out on the right side a fraction of an inch above the dot. **4.** Thread on the button and re-insert the needle a tiny bit below the pencil dot. **5.** On the underside take one small catch-stitch underneath the button -- it won't show -- and then proceed to the next dot without breaking the thread.

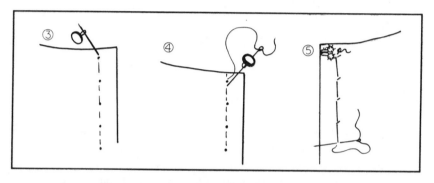

When you come to a place that needs a fastener, lay aside this needle and thread but do not fasten off, and reach for the other threaded needle. Knot the thread and proceed to sew on the snap or hook. Cut off that thread and lay aside. Pick up the other needle and thread and resume sewing on the buttons. Continue in this manner until all the buttons and fasteners are sewn on. This may look tedious, but it is really a very fast business.

Lap the backs and match center back lines. Carefully mark the locations for the thread eyes and the other half of snaps. Sew them in place.

#7 On a tucked-in blouse never sew buttons below the waistline. They make bulging lumps under a smooth-fitting skirt. Substitute snaps or tiny hooks.

#8 You may find ornamental buttons on a chiffon cuff uncomfortable when your arm rests on a hard surface. Snaps can suffice and the uncluttered appearance doesn't compete with other ornaments.

#9 Sometimes plain white buttons, beads and "pearls" can be dyed to match to garment by using the simmering dye bath. Select two beads or buttons to test how they accept the color. Time the procedure. If you achieve the correct color, immerse the entire string. By their nature pearls have a glow; but for buttons, a dull finish looks more attractive.

ZIPPERS

#10 There are many fancy ways to put in a lapped zipper, some of which give a very finished look on the inside of the garment. But who are you trying to impress -- the dry cleaning man? And if your dress is hand-washable ... well, it's pretty hard to find an excuse to display the inside of your costume to your friends. It's better to use a zipper installation that you are completely familiar with, one that gives you the best results in other sewing, as long as it looks very neat from the right side and is as unobtrusive as possible. Your constant goal in sheer sewing is to finish everything so nothing ravels or looks coarse. That includes cloth next to zippers.

#11 In a structured dress such as the ball gown with a fitted bodice, the zipper should be installed by machine for strength. (Always put a hook and eye at an open top.) In a loose-fitting garment put the zipper in by hand or machine, but, of course, the hand installation looks better for chiffon. In a sheer area have the chiffon seam allowance larger than usual so you can effectively manage its raw edges. See ch. 8, #9. Make sure that your disposal of the extra tape at the top looks good from the right side.

#12 For the occasion when a zipper cannot be installed in the back of a garment, the Invisible zipper can often be used successfully in the side seam of a mounted sheer starting about 1/2 in below the armhole as in ch. 8, #11. It lives up to its name of being invisible.

#13 Do not use the above type zipper for a center front or center back installation of a fitted dress or blouse. Its lack of flexibility may cause it to balloon out when you sit.

#14 Before you insert an Invisible zipper whose color isn't quite correct, paint the pull-tab with nail polish to match the fashion fabric.

TUCKS AND LININGS

#15 There is a simple method to prominently display tucks or pleats if they are truly essential to the garment's design. Instead of matching the lining to the sheer, use a much lighter shade of the same color; or use eggshell or a different color altogether. For instance, if your dress is royal blue, you can line it with sky blue, eggshell or green. Each tuck or pleat with its three thicknesses of sheer form a dark stripe of royal blue while the single layer of the sheer join with the lining color to make its own contribution. You may need to line the sleeves with a layer of sheer in the same unusual color as that of the lining.

#16 The covered cord used as a simple edge may appear a lighter color than the other parts of the garment. To overcome this, line the sheer bias covering this way: place the bias strip on the table. On top of it place a strip of bias lining. Lay the cord down the length of the strips and proceed. Always check the effect of lining colors especially when fabrics are pressed closely together.

FITTING

#17 When dressing in a belted shift it is convenient to have the waistline gathers be pre-arranged to your most flattering style. To accomplish this, tie a string around the place you will wear the belt. Have a friend help you arrange the fullness in flattering, random tucks and pin in place immediately above the string. If the lining and sheer are both cut rather generously through the waistline, it's better to arrange the gathers separately. However, you are not trying for a tight fit, but only for control of fullness. Usually, less fullness is required at the center front waist; too much can cause a slight ballooning effect over the chest/diaphragm area unless the sheer fabric is completely flexible. Tack these tucks in place just below the string so that only a small dot of thread appears on the right side, which will be under the belt anyway. The waist will not fit tightly, but the fullness is controlled and placed where it does the most for your figure. Not only can you fasten the belt without fussing with the gathers, but you can relax knowing they will stay in place as you twist and turn.

#18 The so-called fitted sheer garment should be neither tight nor loose; no wrinkles should ever form such places as around the midriff or across the abdomen. If you think it's possible the muslin trial fits too tightly, it probably does. Alter it accordingly.

#19 There may be times when you need to fit only the bodice of the muslin trial dress. Sew it to some sort of skirt that's heavy enough to pull the bodice down to its true location; otherwise, you cannot judge the fit.

HANDWORK

#20 The guide to which kind of stitches to use for handwork depends on how it looks from the outside of the garment. There's no need to spend hours doing some special stitch if the appearance from the right side looks no different from a speedier method.

#21 Normally, when you do any hand-basting, if a knot of thread is left encased in an ordinary garment, you may not like it but you shrug and try to forget about it. With chiffon, organza and some other very sheer fabrics it is quite a different matter. Almost without exception the thread will show from the right side. A good rule to follow is this: don't knot the thread when you baste such a sheer. Take one extra stitch the wrong direction, leaving a tail, and then start sewing. When you remove the bastings, a little careful wiggling will loosen the catch-stitch.

#22 Should a basting be caught in machine stitching, it is imperative that you remove it. Do not pull at the offending thread or you may break the machine stitch. Using your finest little scissors snip it very close to the machine stitch. You can easily remove it by pulling the other end of the basting.

#23 Your old eyebrow tweezers are very useful for removing a basting when only a tiny bit of it protrudes from the cloth.

#24 Many tucks and folds in your sheer creation must be discreetly controlled so that after sponging out or dry cleaning these details are still exactly in place. Thread a needle with matching thread and, inserting it from the wrong side, tack the folds in place so that the stitches neither show from the right side nor hold the cloth down too firmly.

#25 Unless you have your heart set on a black dress, choose some other color for your first garment. It is very difficult to see to do both the machine and hand stitching. The woman who works from 9:00 to 5:00 and must sew on black at night should use a very powerful light. If you can work in daylight hours try to sew on a sunny day and do handwork at a south window. Black is elegant, but this is something to consider.

GOLD NUGGETS

#26 Carefully clip hangnails and file rough places on your fingernails so they won't snag fragile cloth as you handle it.

#27 Wipe the cutting board with a slightly damp Kleenex before you cut out -- particularly important if your last cut-out was a dark fabric and the new is a light color.

#28 When you need to mark your dark colored cloth and the white marker is unobtainable, buy a fingernail whitener pencil. Sharpen it to a needle-like point with the aid of a razor blade, dampen it slightly and use it instead. To remove the white dot, scratch off with your fingernail and/or dampen a Q-Tip swab and twirl it on the spot while you hold a Kleenex underneath.

#29 Do not choose a stripe (woven or printed) to make your first chiffon garment unless your are an expert at cutting and matching. You have enough to handle without this extra challenge.

#30 The details can make or break your costume. If you can make a first-class belt yourself, then do so by all means. If not, have it done professionally. This is no time for economy.

#31 When you put gathering threads in by machine, use fine thread and a fine machine needle so you won't make holes in delicate cloth.

#32 Sometimes you need to change the length of the dress. If you can shorten it enough, simply cut it off and start again; don't bother ripping out something you don't need anyway. Should you need to lengthen, you have to be working with the deep hem to do so. After removing the old hand- stitches carefully, press out the old crease using the correct method you found satisfactory as suggested in ch. 5. If a synthetic fiber still retains the old mark after the vinegar-water solution, you must devise another method of lengthening the garment. The dry cleaner may be able to help you with stubborn creases in silk or rayon that you can't get out. A tell-tale mark always makes the garment look old even when it's quite fashionable otherwise.

LAST-BUT-NOT-LEAST DEPARTMENT

#33 Do you have cousins in another town you can trade clothes with? People with active social lives have done this for years to extend their wardrobes.

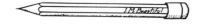

11

CARE AND TRAVEL

It's always a pleasure to finish sewing a special garment, but if it is a sheer -- and especially chiffon -- a sense of supreme satisfaction and amazement may sweep over you. After the last stitch you probably don your creation and look in the mirror admiring your reflection from every possible angle while you move this way and that. You did it! You followed every step, you didn't give up and you finished it. No small thing to be proud of. The joy of seeing yourself in this special garment may be just about more than you can bear. But wait until you wear it in public! If you chose your most flattering color and style, and did your best with the sewing, admiration and compliments will flow your way.

Now it's time for the final touch-up with the iron. And touch-up it is if you followed the suggestions about handling the garment as you proceeded with the cutting and sewing. It's always a good idea to hang the garment on a shaped coat hanger as soon as the neck is finished, and perhaps the sleeves in, to preserve the press. Now your main job is to check the large pieces such as the skirts, and perhaps wide sleeves. Do not go back and give a sharp edge to a yoke, set-in waistband or the like. Overpressing makes your dress look used.

BETWEEN WEARINGS

Hanger

When your garment is in the closet it deserves a shaped hanger of certain specifications. You have several considerations.

The first requirement is that it not be too wide from shoulder tip to shoulder tip. Sometimes the width of a man's suit hanger will make bulges near the top of each sleeve; the only time this isn't a problem is when the garment is sleeveless. You say you are so petite no hanger will do? Here's a possible solution. Go to the boys' suit department (armed with the measurement of the ideal suit-hanger size) and try to buy a good wooden one from an obliging salesperson. Most of us can find one the correct width without too much trouble. We have the added advantage of the new stiff plastic covers to slip over every type from the old wire hanger to the newer tubular ones.

The ideal hanger also approximates your shoulder slope. If you have those lovely sloping shoulders, a very square hanger will cause wrinkles of strain to form across the shoulders under the neck. If you have very square shoulders, the hanger with a definite slope causes your garment to droop sadly with vertical wrinkles in the back, bunches under the arms and an improper hang to the skirt and waist.

Consider the breadth of the shoulder of the hanger from front to back. Only occasionally is the hanger too deep -- it is the thinness you must consider. That's the problem with the wire hanger. However, even some "suit" hangers are too thin. If you have a man's closet to raid, you may be quite surprised at the different shapes of suit hangers. Perhaps you can "avail" yourself of one that's perfect for you.

So, you find a wooden suit hanger that has it all -- width, slope and breadth. But, you see on close inspection that its unfinished wood has tiny rough spots. Although not a problem for a man's suit, such imperfections could snag your fine creation. Ideally, the hanger should also be stain-proof in case you have to hang the garment when it's slightly damp. When you've found the perfect hanger except for this one problem, make it usable by covering it with white plastic or something similar, or even go so far as to sand and paint it.

Never hang the shoulders of a sheer garment on a wire hanger.

Of course, hangers play a completely different role when you have a garment with a halter top. You can sew loops of tape at the waist seam and clothes-pin it to a plastic- covered wire hanger or suspending the side seams from the grippers of a skirt hanger. Ideally, you can loop the halter neck around the hook of the hanger; but it may work better to let the bodice hang down over the skirts.

In the Closet

Perhaps you have read that Mamie Eisenhower used a spare bedroom in the White House as a closet for her gowns. They hung on racks with plenty of space between so bouffant skirts could be fluffed out and nothing would get crushed. How we envy her all that space! Most of us must make do with the space available in our inadequate closets.

Unless you have many different circles of friends, your sheer garment may hang in the closet a while between wearings. It behooves you to do right by it when you put it there and then see that later you don't push it around roughly. Simply observe the usual good practices of the closet-wise: adjust the shoulders carefully on the correct hanger, close zippers and fasten the buttons. Arrange the sleeves to hang down without twisting and make sure pocket flaps are in place. Smooth skirts so they fall properly. Never crush it against other garments. If you must let it hang a long time between wearings, cover it with a large, very lightweight dust-cover. Do not fold it up for storage and never keep it in the basement. (Do you have an attic? Install a temporary hanging rack and use it to suspend the covered garment. The dry air will not harm your gown.)

With this careful attention your synthetic costume will seldom if ever need pressing, although a rayon or silk gown may have a few long soft creases in the skirt or sleeves that need your attention. If you cut your garment absolutely on the grain as described in ch. 5 and let the dress hang before marking the hem, it will take such careful handling in the closet without losing its shape.

GENERAL CARE

Accidents

You wear your perfect creation to the special event. Just as you hoped, it is exactly right for the occasion and you think you look just great. (So does everyone else.) Then someone bumps your arm and food and drink go all over the front.

If your gown is silk or rayon, wipe off what you can. Then you must judge if water will hurt any interfacing, etc. If you shrunk everything it probably won't. Then handle as you would any drycleanable fabric. If this accident happened in the daytime, take the garment to the drycleaners that day; if at night, the next day. Promptness is important.

Synthetic fabric is easy. If you planned washing your garment and treated each item involved in the construction of it accordingly, simply go at once to the powder room and while you hold a towel or such underneath, sponge out the offending spots according to the spill as you would any washable fiber. Was it red wine? Promptly treat it with club soda. When you're finished try to borrow a hand-held hair dryer from your host(ess), dry the fabric as best you can and return to the party. You will probably want to wash the garment when you get home.

General Washing

When an entire synthetic garment needs washing, you may sponge it out by hand using the manufacturer's directions on the bottle of Delicare or Woolite. Use fabric softener in the last rinse water. Synthetic fiber is really quite tough. You may treat any spots with your usual products and blood spots with a bar of Ivory soap and cold water. Of course, it's easier to put the whole thing in the automatic washer and quite safe if you planned for it. Treat the spots, set the machine on DELICATE wash and rinse. Again, use special detergent and use fabric softener in the last rinse cycle as suggested in ch. 5.

What about those combination affairs such as TWO LAYERS OF CHIFFON -- can they be machine-washed, too? Yes, if you follow the preceding suggestions AND if you made the dress as outlined. Did you handle the pleat creases with the tiny back-stitches? Cut the layers separately, absolutely on the straight of grain and mount carefully? Follow the other systems? If so, you may machine wash.

Drying

The best way to dry your synthetic garment is in the automatic dryer. Put the wet garment in the dryer along with something like a towel (or other clothes) and set it on the temperature for synthetics. Remove from the dryer the instant it's ready -- or a few seconds before -- and hang it properly on its hanger as described earlier. Work like the wind so no wrinkles will form in the warm cloth. Hang where the air can circulate around it and when cool, examine for creases. Here's something to remember about washing and wrinkles in your synthetic garment. If it goes into the washer deeply wrinkled, it comes out of the dryer wrinkled. It's the nature of the brute. Wonderful as polyester is, it won't magically lose its creases as it goes through the washing business. If for some reason you have such a wrinkled garment and you know its history, that it's really clean but badly mussed, press it before you wash it. (Remember, no mashing down those special places you want to have that soft appearance.) That way, when you take it out of the dryer, you may hang it up and it's ready to wear when dry. If, however, you are uncertain what's happened to it in the past, examine it closely for spots in the usual places, treat them and then wash it. We all know it's not a good idea to press in soil of any kind. After it comes from the dryer, hang it properly and when dry, press it with a warm iron. It's unlikely, but you may have to use vinegar-water solution to get out some deep creases.

GOING PLACES

We live in the age of constant travel. It is not uncommon to go to another city to attend a party or wedding. How shall you transport your special sheer creation? You fear wrinkles caused by packing will necessitate your trying to find an ironing board and iron (usually unreliable) upon arrival. A dress that is even part rayon will not travel well no matter how careful you try to be. You will have to press it when you arrive. Pure silk is a much better traveler. Polyester is your best traveling companion. However you travel, an inflatable plastic hanger is most useful. It lies flat in your suitcase until needed.

By Plane

At the last minute just before you go to the airport, fold the dress very loosely including lots of tissue paper to soften the folds and place it in a large paper shopping bag (not plastic which has no body). Hand-carry it on to the plane and stow it under the seat in front of you or on the floor between your feet. You can put it in the overhead compartment but it's very hard to insist nothing is put on top of it. If you want to check the garment along with the rest of your baggage, put it in its own hard-side luggage -- and then pray your luggage isn't lost. When you arrive, hang up the sheer at once.

By Car

When you travel by car everything is much easier. Put the garment in a lightweight garment bag (or a plastic leaf bag) and put it in the trunk or back seat. You may fold it at the waist if the car is small or the garment long. If you must suspend from a bar across the back seat, drape with something to protect from the sun and covetous eyes. Further, it's no problem to take your own iron, which you are completely familiar with, and an ironing blanket to use for any slight touch-ups when you reach your destination. Hang the garment up at once upon arrival.

Wear your creation every chance you get. Enjoy it!

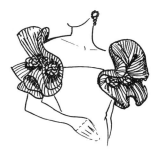

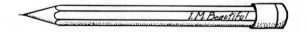

ADDITIONAL INFORMATION

Pictured are two McCall's patterns which you will find helpful if you don't have suitable patterns for linings in your collection.

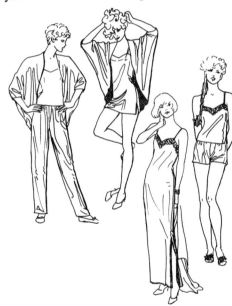

McCall's number 4608, which comes in sizes X-Small, Small, Medium and Large, has to be one of your best buys with patterns for six garments -- nightgown, tunic, camisole, pants, shorts, plus and interesting jacket. Consider the pants as a liner for the very full trouser.

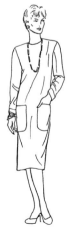

McCall's number 4450, found in the STITCH 'N SAVE section, can be helpful for the shift. It comes in sizes A (8-10) and B (12, 14, 16).

more →

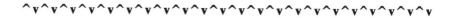

Your fabric store manager can order cloth from the following firms. They do NOT deal with the general public.

ROBERT KAUFMAN CO., INC.
2135 West 132nd Street
Los Angeles, CA 90061
1-800-877-2066

This company produces a chiffon, Triple Sheer, made from high-twist yarns, that has a fine hand and drapes beautifully.

EASTERN SILK CO.
55 West 39th Street
New York, NY 10018
(212) 730-1300

This firm deals in pure silk.

GLICK TEXTILES
1901 Capitol
Houston, TX 77003
1-800-231-7246

This company is a boon to the smaller store that cannot order thousands of yards but wants to supply the customer with quality merchandise.

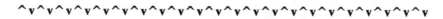

To send your material off to be pleated before you sew the garment, first sew together the panels required to fit the area when the pleats are closed and then hem. Various styles of pleats are available. For information send SASE to

SAN FRANCISCO PLEATING CO.
425 2nd Street
San Francisco, CA 94107
(415) 982-3003

INDEX

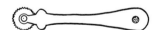

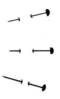

Order this book for a friend who sews.

Please send _____ copies of SEW CHIFFON and OTHER SHEERS to:

Name_____

Street_____

State_____Zip_____Pho_____

VISA#_____Exp. Date_____

MasterCard#_____Exp. Date_____

I enclose $19.95 plus $2.50 for shipping and handling for each book. TN residents also include sales tax.

Authorized Signature_____

Send to: B. L. Frame Publishing

PO Box 1379

Lebanon TN   37088

If book is to be sent to another address, please fill out:

Name_____

Address_____

City_____State_____Zip_____

Cut on dotted line

To:

From:

We'll enclose this with the book.

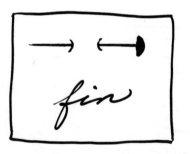